THE DALY DISH

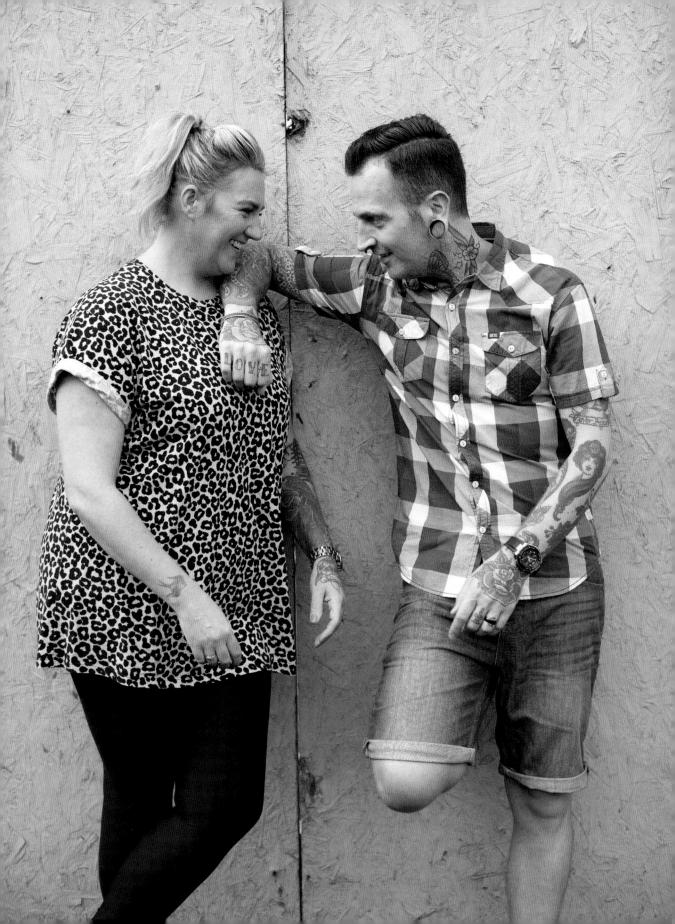

THE
DALY
DISH

100 Masso Slimming Meals
FOR EVERY DAY

GINA DALY AND MR DISH

GILL BOOKS

Gill Books

Hume Avenue

Park West

Dublin 12

www.gillbooks.ie

Gill Books is an imprint of M.H. Gill and Co.

© Gina Daly 2020

Mister Dish's Dishes recipes © Karol Daly 2020

978 07171 8649 5

Designed by www.grahamthew.com

Photography by Leo Byrne

Photo of airfryer on p. 4 © Shutterstock

Food styling by Charlotte O'Connell, assisted by Claire Wilkinson

Edited by Susan McKeever

Proofread by Jane Rogers

Indexed by Eileen O'Neill

Printed and Bound in Germany by Firmengruppe APPL

This book is typeset in 10 on 14 point Sentinel Light.
The paper used in this book comes from the wood pulp of managed forests.
For every tree felled, at least one tree is planted, thereby renewing natural resources.

A CIP catalogue record for this book is available from
the British Library.

10 9 8 7 6

ABOUT THE AUTHORS

Gina and Karol Daly live in County Meath with their two children.
Gina is an illustrator who, with Karol, runs The Bitch Box, an
online greeting card company that shares their sense of humour.
Working together, cooking together and having the craic together,
there's never a dull moment in the Dish household.

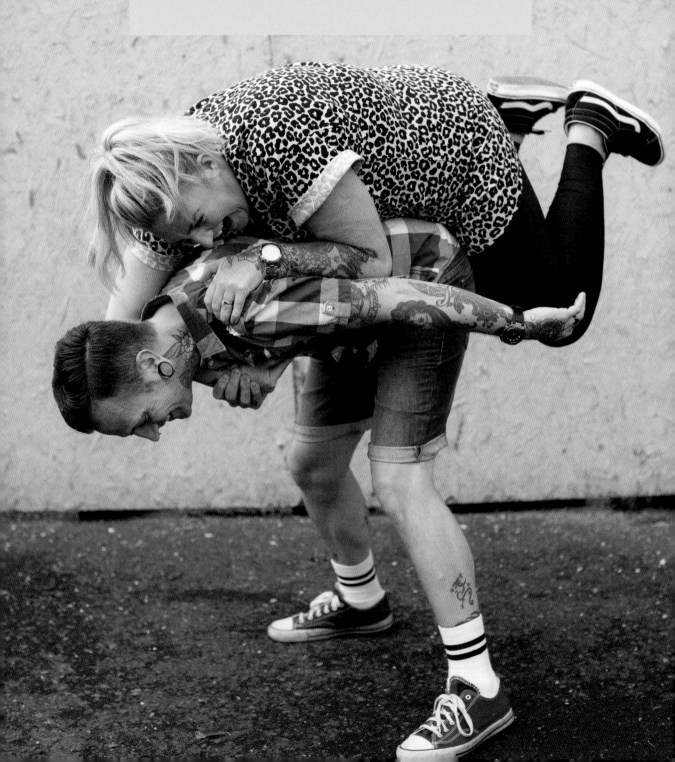

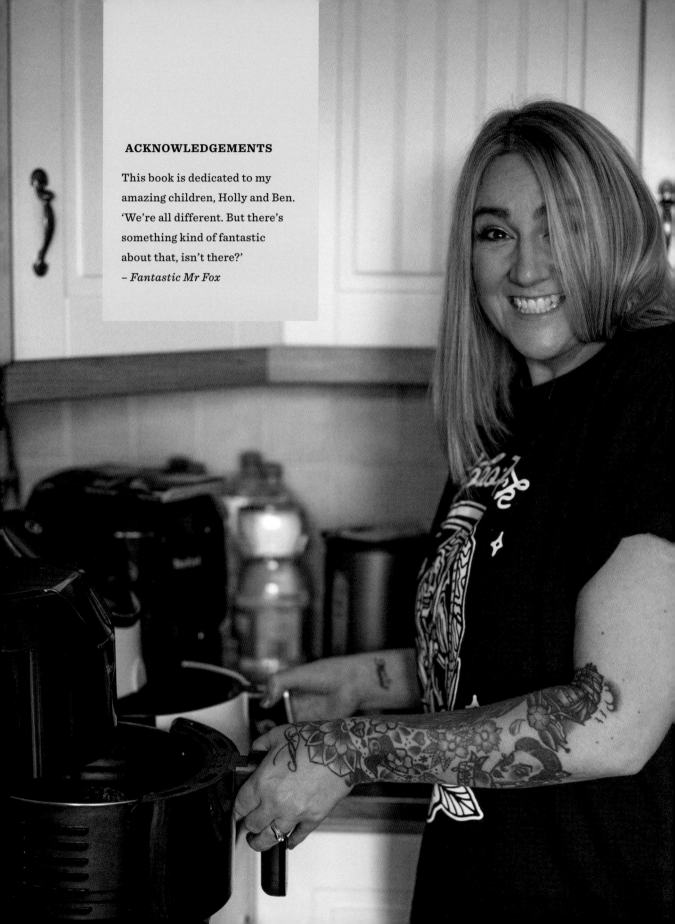

ACKNOWLEDGEMENTS

This book is dedicated to my amazing children, Holly and Ben. 'We're all different. But there's something kind of fantastic about that, isn't there?'
– *Fantastic Mr Fox*

CONTENTS

Introduction 1

The Airfryer 4

Shopping List and Bits 6

Dishy Dinners 9

Ask Me Airfryer 43

Fake Makes 61

Savage Snacks 93

Saucy Sauces 133

Mister Dish's Dishes 145

Masso Mia 169

Deadly & Delicious 193

Index 211

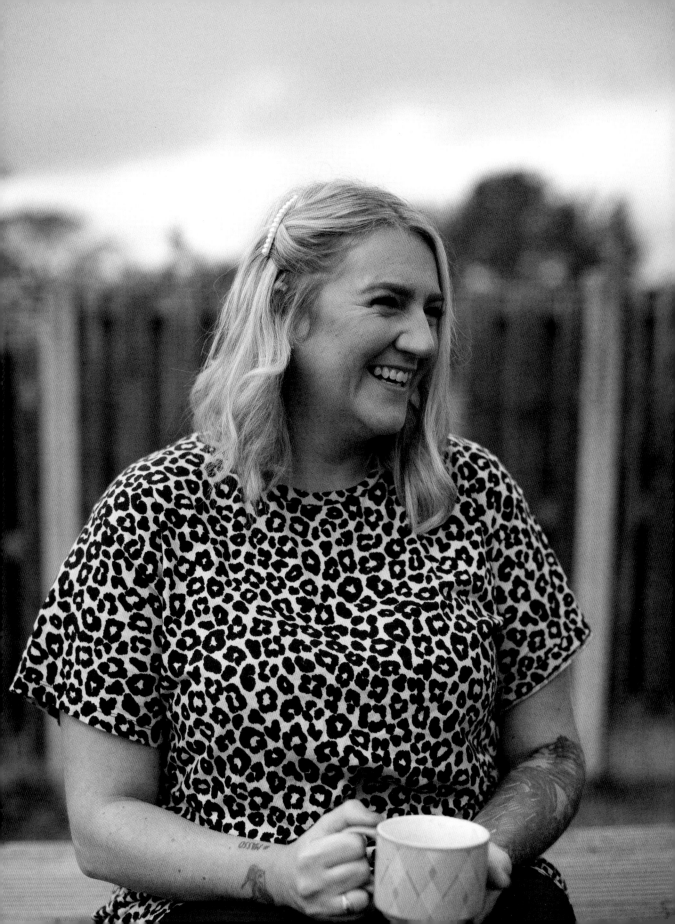

INTRODUCTION

Howya, my name is Gina and you're welcome to my book. I can't actually believe I have typed those words! But I have, and if you are reading this it must be real.

I am a busy mam of two, living in County Meath with my little divils, Holly and Ben, and my deadly husband Karol, the man who made me the woman I am today. Now, I know what you are all thinking, you don't need a fella to make you who you are and, yes, you are right, but without his support, encouragement and absolute love for me (no matter what I look like), he has given me the confidence I have always struggled to find.

Karol and I started our life together in what can only be described as a whirlwind. We met, got engaged two weeks later, and then got married six months after that, as you do! On our first date he changed his name on my phone to 'My Hubbie' and said that's what he was going to be. I was weak! I still haven't changed it 12 years later.

Like most couples starting out, we very quickly became comfortable in each other's company and ate out a lot, got takeaway every second night and rarely made a home-cooked meal; and if we did, it was always convenience food as we had such busy work schedules.

Fast-forward seven years, two small kids and a lot of shite food, we both found ourselves overweight and unhealthy. I suffered really badly with gallstones, so had to have surgery to have them removed and in the few weeks of recovery I lost a lot of weight from eating a low-fat diet.

Despite the way it came about, I felt so much better in myself once I lost the weight. My skin was healthier and my clothes were looser, so I knew I wanted to keep going as that feeling was great. However, slowly but surely the shite food crept back in and the weight started to go back on! So, enough was enough. I joined a local slimming club. This was the start of it all for me. I lost four stone in four months and was delighted with my life. I was down to the slimmest I had been since I was a teenager and was able to buy clothes from all the high street shops and ... with all my healthy eating and cooking, Karol dropped an incredible four stone too.

I left the group but continued cooking and eating 'all to plan' and then ... well, then it just became boring. I found myself eating the same dinners every week because I had no imagination. It even got to the stage where I was looking for any excuse to have a takeaway. I did my best to keep my meals good, but I was snacking like a mad thing on crisps and chocolate in between because I wasn't getting satisfied from my dinners. I just wasn't enjoying it anymore. I needed the junk. I needed the bad stuff. I was cracking!

Now, can you guess what happened next?

Well, I'll tell you, Mary. I piled the four feckin' stone back on. I just didn't give a shite and every Monday was my 'I'll start today' day.

Meanwhile, Karol was out running every day, doing his weights and eating all the 'rabbit food', as I called it. It just wasn't for me any more, but at the same time I wanted to be healthier, so therein lay my dilemma.

Then one day, as if I got a hoof up the arse from Satan himself, it all clicked! Now, I was no chef, and I certainly never claimed to have a great imagination when it came to meals, but I realised I could eat the food I wanted to eat, and with a few tweaks here and there I could make them healthy and low-fat. Sure Jaysus it was like I had won the food lottery.

So I set up an Instagram account called 'The Daly Dish' (I'm Gina Daly, so see what I did there? Yes, I'm an actual genius) and started to log my meals to keep myself on track. Within a few short months I'd lost three stone by eating what felt like a treat every night of the week! The more I cooked the better I became at turning traditionally high-fat meals into healthier versions of themselves.

However, while I was 'fixing' the outside I still had a massive hurdle to overcome.

Fixing the inside.

While losing the weight was great because I was getting healthier, my mindset was far from healthy. I was so obsessively focused on the number on the scales and how I would feel if I reached 'target', I didn't realise that no matter what size I got to I would never really truly be happy. Why? Because I didn't really love myself or even like the person who was looking back at me in the mirror. I picked her apart. Tore her to shreds. Criticised every lump and bump and wished she looked different or she didn't have those jiggly thighs or that fat on her back. I was so hard on myself.

In 2018 myself and Karol went on our first proper holiday on our own without the kids to Ibiza. I had said to myself, if I lose three stone for this holiday, 'I'll be happy'. I lost the three stone and off we went. I sat at the pool, surrounded by what to me looked like models in string bikinis, and there's me in me big muumuu all covered up. I was nervous to get in the pool in case people judged me or thought I had fat legs or a fat arse, but as I sat and looked around I noticed that not one person, not one, was looking at me. Not one single person would have cared if I had a turnip for a head! And why? Because they were all too worried about what they looked like themselves to notice anyone else. I could see girls uncomfortably adjusting their tops and pulling down the sides of their bikinis and popping on sarongs to walk to the pool and it was in that moment in my life, after 37 years, I realised that I was the only person who cared what I looked like.

So, I whipped off the muumuu; now it took a few vinos for the Dutch courage, I won't lie, but Karol took my hand and we walked together around the pool, legs out, arse out, all my giblets in full motion, and not one single person batted an eyelid! Not one fecker and, to be honest, I was kind of raging because I wanted to be proved right. I wanted to prove I was being judged, but I wasn't. I sat down and kept looking to see who was staring at me and, again, no one was! And that was it. That was the 'lightbulb' moment. That was when I started to turn my insecurities into a strength. I tore down that wall of negativity and started to rebuild it as a wall of positivity, a wall that no one would ever break down, not even me.

So now, it doesn't matter what I weigh. It doesn't matter if I'm a 10 or a 20. What matters is how I feel in myself, and feeling confident and sexy in your own body, regardless of weight or size, is an actual superpower.

I don't look back now on old photos and hate the person I see. I remember why she was so happy at that moment in time and that she is the girl that got me to where I am today, but I've learned to mind her a little better cause she's masso!

So here, I present to you 90 of my favourite recipes that have really helped me on my journey to becoming a healthier me. And, as if that weren't enough, there are 10 bonus recipes from Karol, aka Mr Dish (I gave him his own chapter). He's become quite the cook over the years, too!

All our recipes are fun, quick and easy to make and can be enjoyed by the whole family. We hope you enjoy them as much as we do. (P.S. You will see that I use the word 'masso' or '#masso' from time to time – that means 'deadly', 'fab' or 'gorgeous' in the Daly household.)

THE AIRFRYER

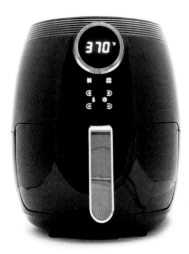

This baby, which sounds a bit like some kind of spaceship, plays a massive role in my day-to-day cooking. I genuinely think I would be lost without it – it was definitely the best purchase I ever made. Now, while it's not essential to have one, the fact is we all love a bit of convenience and when time is of the essence this little beauty will save so much of that.

WHAT IS AN AIRFRYER? LET ME TELL YOU

This electrical wonder is basically a small tabletop convection oven. It works the same way as your fan oven does, cooking food by blowing hot air down around the food, but in a smaller capacity, therefore it cooks food up to 25 per cent faster. It also doesn't need to be preheated, so it's super convenient. It also uses very little oil to cook the food, so you get the wonderful crispness of fried food but with a lot less fat.

THINGS YOU SHOULD KNOW BEFORE PURCHASING

There are many different brands out there and, in my experience, I haven't come across a bad one yet. The main thing you need to look for is the capacity. There will be various sizes starting from a 1.5 litre (possibly smaller) up to a 5 litre plus, so it's important to choose the right size for your family. I have a 4.2 litre one and it will cook enough food for up to six people. You can pick one up for about €80 online or in an electrical shop so it won't break the bank.

ARE THEY NOT ONLY FOR CHIPS?

This is the question I get asked all the time and the simple answer is absolutely not! It is so much more than a chip maker. I literally cook everything in it, or should I say, everything that will fit in it. From your veg to your whole chicken, you can do anything! It will bake bread, muffins and cookies and it will also cook bacon and sausages, mushrooms, omelettes, crispy chicken; Jaysus, the list goes on and on! If it fits inside, it will cook it.

The trick to keep the food super crispy is not to overfill the basket, so while you might have the urge to shove a rake of chips to feed the nation in there, keeping the quantities small and doing them in batches will get you better results. If I'm making food for the family in batches, I leave the first batch to one side in a bowl and then, when the second batch is done, I throw the first batch back in and it will heat it up! Simple!

HANDY THINGS TO KNOW

You can use things like tinfoil and greaseproof paper inside the airfryer too, as long as they don't block the vents and stop the air flowing around. It won't blow up, don't worry. Just be sure you don't let the greaseproof paper touch the element or it might start to burn.

You can also pop in baking tins, or muffin moulds, etc., if you're using it for baking.

HOW DO YOU CLEAN IT?

The majority of the baskets are dishwasher-safe, so you can fire them in after every use. My advice is to give it a rinse or a light scrub after each use. Even though you use little oil, the fan blows hot air around and any oil will also blow around and can cause a build-up on the sides. If you leave it too long it can become tougher to get rid of, so just keep on top of it.

WHAT OIL DO YOU USE?

It's best to use an oil with a high smoke or burning point. I use two-calorie rapeseed oil that can take a high heat before it starts to burn. Using an oil with a low smoke point will burn into your appliance with the high heat of the airfryer and leave a film that's very hard to remove and, in some cases, will void your warranty.

The same applies to your non-stick pots and pans. If you are using an oil with a low smoke point and you find the non-stick is not non-stick any more, this is the reason why! Check the labels and know your oils.

A NOTE ON OTHER APPLIANCES

Some of the recipes in the book call for a waffle maker; one calls for a doughnut maker. These may sound like luxury items to some people, but they are really very handy to come by. You'll pick them up relatively cheaply in some of the bigger supermarkets, or in your local electrical shop. And once you've seen how handy they are for whipping up impressive home-made waffles and doughnuts, you'll never look back!

SHOPPING LIST AND BITS

Being prepared is so important when you are embarking on any weight loss/ healthy eating journey. Having time-saving essentials in the press will be your lifesaver, especially if you have a busy day or week ahead. This list of store cupboard essentials will help you get started and give you all you need to start making deadly dishes. Even the simplest of ingredients can lend to a wholesome, filling meal and will save you reaching for the goodies.

So, whether it's beans on toast or a full-blown fake make, I've got ya covered with these handy few bits that will jazz up any meal.

TINNED BITS:
- Tomatoes
- Baked beans
- Spaghetti hoops
- Mushy peas
- Chickpeas
- Kidney beans
- Sweetcorn
- Light coconut milk
- Mustard powder

BOTTLES AND JARS:
- Passata
- Soy sauce
- Hot sauce
- Buffalo hot sauce
- BBQ sauce
- Worcestershire sauce
- Easy/lazy garlic
- Easy/lazy chillis
- Black bean concentrate
- Sriracha sauce
- Dijon mustard
- Low-fat vinaigrette
- Jalapeño peppers
- Gherkins
- Light Caesar dressing
- Lighter than light mayo
- Peanut butter

STOCK CUBES:
My everyday essential, the base for most of my sauces and soups. I prefer stock pots but cubes are just as good.
- Vegetable
- Beef
- Chicken
- Herb
- Red wine

DRIED BITS:
- Pasta (all shapes)
- Rice
- Couscous
- Vermicelli noodles
- Egg noodles
- Sesame seeds (deadly for garnishing)
- Instant mashed potato
- Savoury yeast flakes (available in health-food shops)
- Panko breadcrumbs

HERBS AND SPICES

These are the main herbs and spices I use in nearly all my dishes. I can literally make anything with these bad boys.

- Smoked paprika
- Paprika
- Garlic powder
- Ground ginger
- Lemon pepper (use sea salt mixed with black pepper if you can't find this)
- Chilli powder
- Mixed herbs
- Sage
- Ground cumin
- Cinnamon
- Curry powder
- Chinese five spice powder
- Sea salt
- Black pepper

BREAD AND WRAPS

- High-fibre wholemeal bread
- Wholemeal pitta bread
- Wholemeal wraps

OTHER BITS:

- Low-calorie spray oil (I use rapeseed two-calorie spray)
- Porridge oats
- Baking powder
- Frozen petits pois
- Cornflour
- Cocoa powder
- Vanilla essence
- Sweetener (any granulated type)

- Vinegar
- Zero-calorie syrups
- Zero-sugar cola
- Zero-sugar orange
- Zero-sugar cordial

Keeping your fridge stocked with lots of fruit and veg is also essential to get you from day to day. Bulking up your plate with extra veggies is a great way to exercise portion control. You are getting the benefits of the good stuff while reducing your carb intake by putting less pasta, rice or potatoes on your plate. You also won't get a bloated feeling, common after carb overload.

If you are a grazer, having fruits like watermelon, strawberries, raspberries, blueberries, etc. is a great way to have a nice little snack and also get that sweet hit at the same time; if you want something a little more filling, stock up on fat-free yoghurts or flavoured quark and throw your berries in on top!

DISHY DINNERS

Terrifically Tasty

BEEF SATAY

This is the perfect weekend treat. No, scrap that – it's an any-day-of-the-week treat and I guarantee you will have it more than once in the week! One of my favourite dishes is a good satay. Only problem is that it's loaded with calories, so I made it my mission to make a satay just as good, no, actually better than I could get from my local takeout. So here it is, in all its glory, my terrifically tasty beef satay.

SERVES 2

Low-calorie spray oil

Veg – use whichever veg you prefer, I like the following: mangetout, green beans, scallions, fresh red chilli

2 tbsp dark soy sauce

2 lean beef medallions

280g rice (whichever kind you prefer)

1 fresh red chilli, sliced, to garnish (optional)

For the satay sauce:

1 can zero-sugar cola

1–2 tbsp peanut butter (depending on how peanutty you want it to taste)

1–2 tbsp curry powder

1 tsp garlic granules

1 tsp paprika

Chilli flakes (add to your own taste, I like mine spicy)

½ tsp ginger (optional), I use the squeezable one in a tube

3–4 drops Worcestershire sauce

Salt to taste (optional as the soy is very salty)

1 Heat up your wok with a little spray oil, throw in the veg with the soy sauce and cook until tender but still retaining a little 'bite'. Remove from the wok and transfer to a plate nearby.

2 Next up, add all the sauce ingredients into your wok. Stir everything together and bring to the boil until thickened.

3 If you need to loosen it, add a dash of water.

4 Next, fry up your steaks on a separate, non-stick frying pan. I like mine rare so give only a quick blast on each side. Remove from the pan when cooked to your taste and leave to rest for a few minutes.

5 Return the veg to the wok and stir into the sauce.

6 Now get your rice ready, divide between two plates/bowls, slice up your steak and place strips on top of the rice, then pour over your sauce and veg, topping with some sliced chilli if you like. Enjoy every bite – if you're anything like me you'll lick the plate clean!

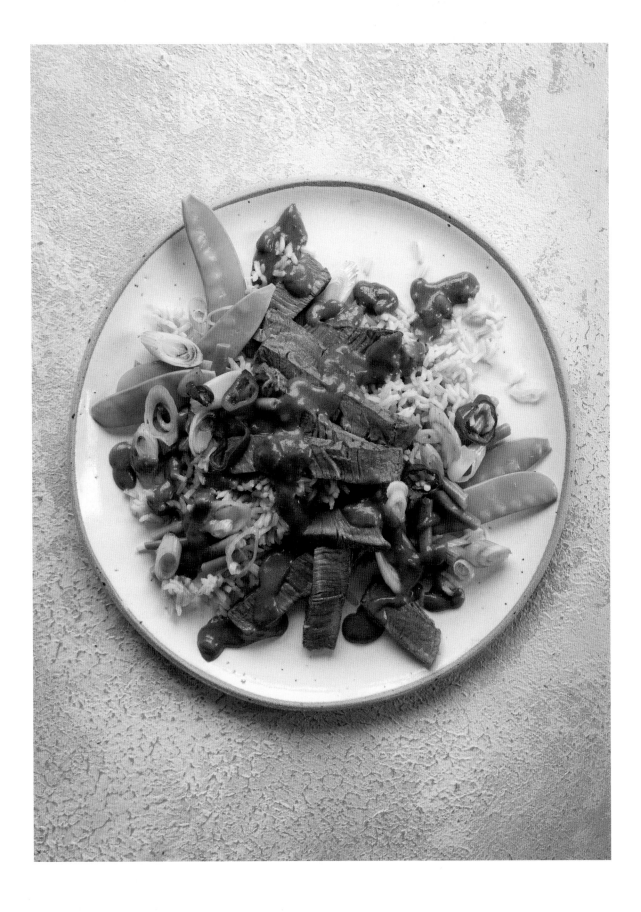

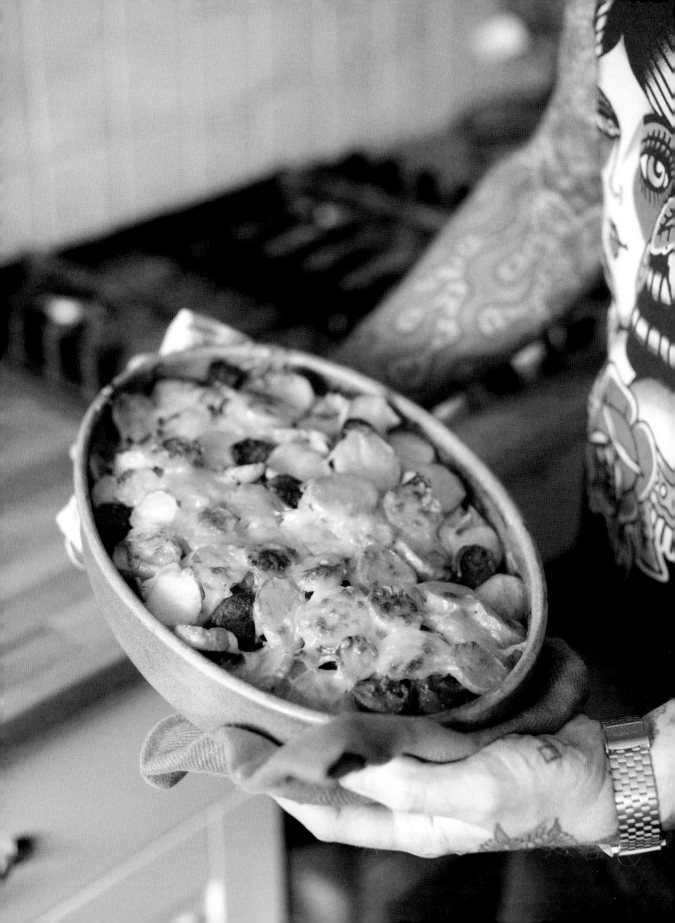

Chicken, Leek and
CHORIZO PIE

I have been making this dish for years and would have normally made the sauce with lots of cream, but I adjusted the ingredients to make it less calorific while being able to keep the amazing flavour of the broth. It's comforting and so easy to make and while it's not technically a pie, I'm calling it a pie. Preparation basically consists of layering up ingredients as in a lasagne, but using potatoes as the pasta layer.

SERVES 4

4 chicken fillets, chopped

100g chorizo, sliced

350g mushrooms, chopped

2 large leeks, well rinsed and chopped

500g boiled baby potatoes, sliced thinly

15g Grana Padano, grated

300ml hot chicken stock

1 tsp garlic powder

1 tsp smoked paprika

3 light cheese singles, torn into pieces

80g low-fat Cheddar cheese, grated

1 Preheat the oven to 200°C.

2 Take half the chicken, chorizo, mushrooms and leeks and scatter evenly over the bottom of a Pyrex dish.

3 Layer half the boiled potatoes evenly across the top of the chicken, chorizo and veg, then sprinkle half the Grana Padano over the top of the potatoes.

4 Repeat the chicken, chorizo, leek and mushroom layer using up the second half of the ingredients, topping again with a layer of the spuds and a sprinkle of the cheese.

5 Prepare your chicken stock in a mixing jug, then add the garlic powder, smoked paprika and the torn-up cheese singles. Give it a good mix until the cheese has melted into the stock.

6 Pour this over the top of the 'pie', sprinkle the Cheddar cheese on top, cover with foil and pop it into your preheated oven for 30–40 minutes, removing the foil for the last 10 minutes to allow the cheese to go golden brown.

7 Once it's ready serve in warm bowls and ladle over that delicious broth – the flavour of this is incredible.

Chicken

ENCHILADAS

We love a big feast and these are just what's needed after a long day at work. Comforting, bursting with flavour and ready in no time. Here's my take on this Mexican beauty.

SERVES 4

Low-calorie spray oil

1 onion, sliced

1 red pepper, deseeded and sliced

250g chopped mushrooms

4 chicken fillets, chopped into bite-sized pieces

2 tbsp sweet chilli sauce

2 tbsp buffalo hot sauce

4 wholemeal high-fibre wraps

60g reduced-fat Cheddar cheese, grated

10 green jalapeños

Fresh coriander to garnish (optional)

For the enchilada sauce:

1 x 500g carton of passata

1 tsp chilli powder

1 tsp smoked paprika

2 tbsp buffalo hot sauce

1 tsp soy sauce

½ tsp garlic powder

100ml beef stock

3 slices light cheese singles, torn into pieces

2 tbsp juice from jar of jalapeños

½ chicken stock pot

1 Preheat the oven to 200°C.

2 First make the enchilada sauce. Put all the sauce ingredients in a small pot over a medium heat. Stir until all the ingredients are blended and the cheese has melted and is smooth. Remove from the heat and leave to one side.

3 Grab a frying pan and on a medium heat fry off onion, pepper and mushrooms until softened. Remove from the pan and leave to one side.

4 Wipe out the pan with some kitchen paper, spray on a little more oil and fry the chicken pieces until browned. Add the sweet chilli sauce and cook for 2–3 minutes until golden and sticky, then add in the hot sauce and stir to coat the chicken evenly.

5 Add the veg back in and toss with the chicken.

6 Next lay out the wraps, spread 1 tbsp of the enchilada sauce on each wrap, then add even amounts of the chicken and veg to each and roll up the wraps.

7 Grab a deep baking tray and lay out the wraps, folded side down.

8 Pour the remaining sauce evenly over the enchilada wraps, sprinkle with the Cheddar cheese and scatter over the jalapeños.

9 Pop into the preheated oven for 15–20 mins until the cheese has melted and is golden brown. Remove, sprinkle over the coriander if using, and serve immediately.

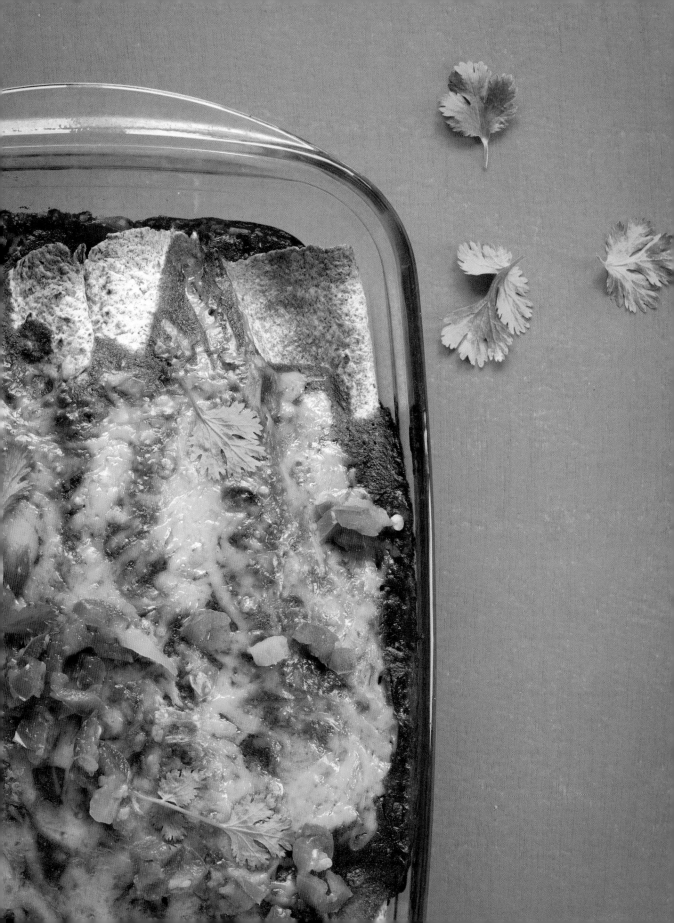

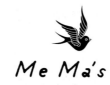

Me Ma's

CHICKEN CURRY

Remember when you used to come in from school and the gaff would be leppin with the smell of your ma's dinner? I'll never forget it, and on the coldest of days she used to make this masso curry. So comforting and brings back so many lovely memories. Even if she used to eat the head off me for the state of my room when I got in the door.

SERVES 4

4 large chicken fillets

800ml chicken stock

2 tbsp medium curry powder

1 tbsp turmeric

2 tsp chilli powder

1 small apple, peeled, cored and chopped

6 cloves roasted garlic (see page 170)

100ml light cream

½ tsp ground ginger

1 tsp garlic powder

1 large onion, chopped

½ tsp Chinese five spice powder

1 tsp white wine vinegar

1 tsp sweetener

1 tsp cornflour (optional)

150g frozen petits pois

360g dried long-grain rice

1 My mother used to always boil her chicken for the curry, so that's the way I like to do it. Put the whole breasts in a large pot of boiling water and let them cook away for 15–20 minutes until cooked through. Remove from the water, then use a couple of forks to shred it up (my fave) or chop it into chunks.

2 Now make the sauce. Put the chicken stock in a hot wok, add in the curry powder, the turmeric (this will add a lovely yellow colour to the curry) and the chilli powder and stir until well mixed.

3 Crush the apple and garlic in a pestle and mortar, and add to the wok.

4 Bring up the heat and let it cook away for 10 minutes. At this point I stick a hand blender straight into the wok to break down and smooth the apple and garlic.

5 Add in the cream, ginger, garlic powder, chopped onion, Chinese five spice, white wine vinegar and sweetener, give it a good stir and bring to the boil for 3–4 minutes. Add in your chicken, then reduce the heat and let simmer for 10–15 minutes until the sauce thickens. If the sauce is not as thick as you would like, mix the cornflour with a few drops of water and gradually stir into the curry until it thickens. Finally stir in the petits pois and stir until they are heated through.

6 Prep your rice and serve it up with the curry in warmed bowls. This is great for a batch cook and will freeze really well too.

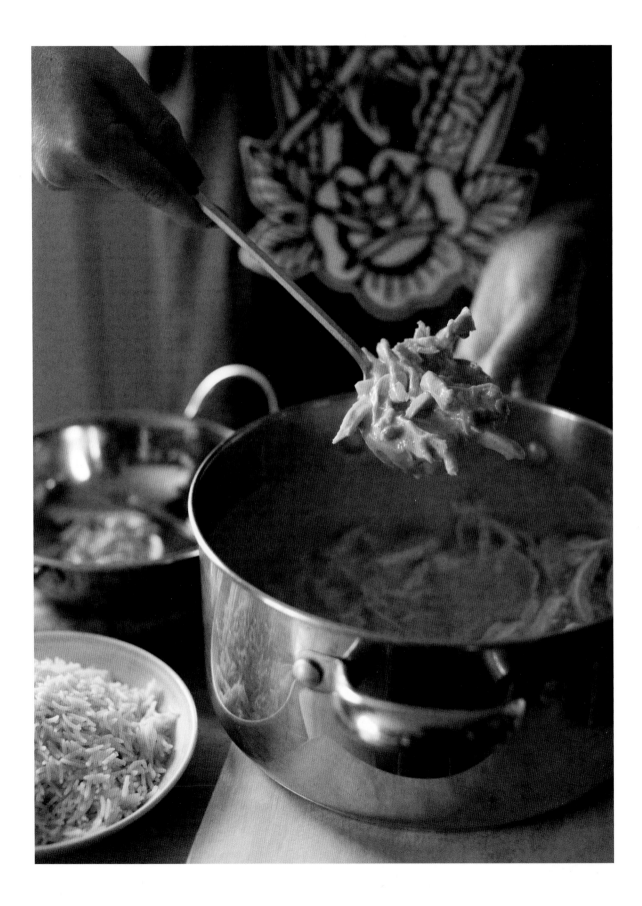

Cheesy
CHICKRIZO PASTA

The perfect combo of chicken and chorizo make this a dish you'll want to make over and over again.

SERVES 4

300g dried spaghetti or pasta of choice

Low-calorie spray oil

4 chicken fillets, chopped

1 tsp lemon pepper

300ml chicken stock

50g chorizo, chopped

6 light cheese singles, torn

1 tsp smoked paprika

1 tsp garlic powder

15g Parmesan cheese, grated (plus extra to serve)

1 First you are going to prep the pasta, so in a large pan bring some salted water to the boil and add in the pasta. Cook until al dente, drain and put to one side.

2 Spray a wok with some oil and lash the chicken and the lemon pepper in. Cook over a medium heat until the chicken is browned.

3 Now pour in the chicken stock and let that simmer for a minute or two.

4 Add in the chopped chorizo and the cheese singles, bring up the heat and stir like a mad thing until the cheese blends and melts into the sauce.

5 Add in the smoked paprika and garlic powder along with the Parmesan cheese.

6 Bring down the heat and let this wok of massoness simmer until the sauce starts to thicken, then toss in the pasta and stir until every strand is well coated. Serve in bowls with extra Parmesan, if wanted.

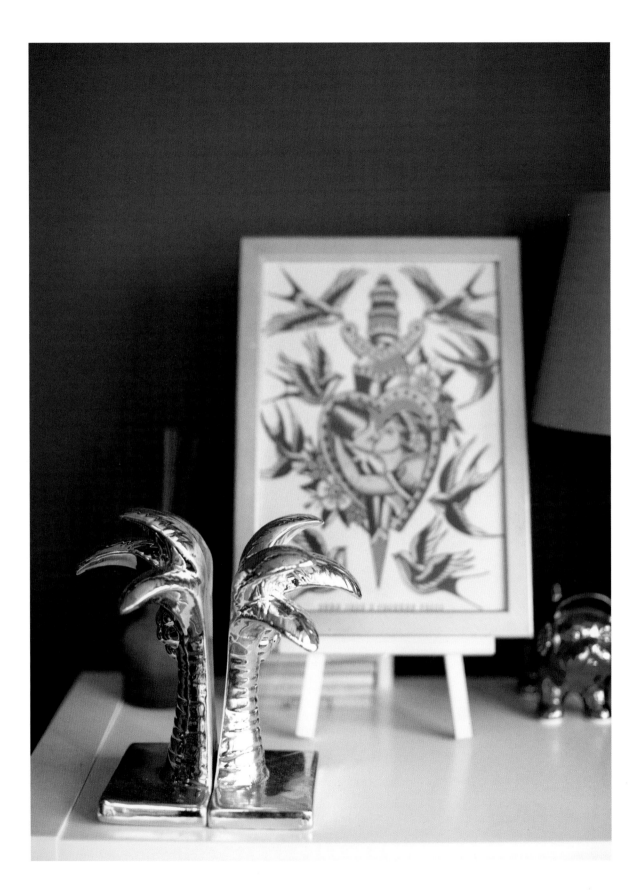

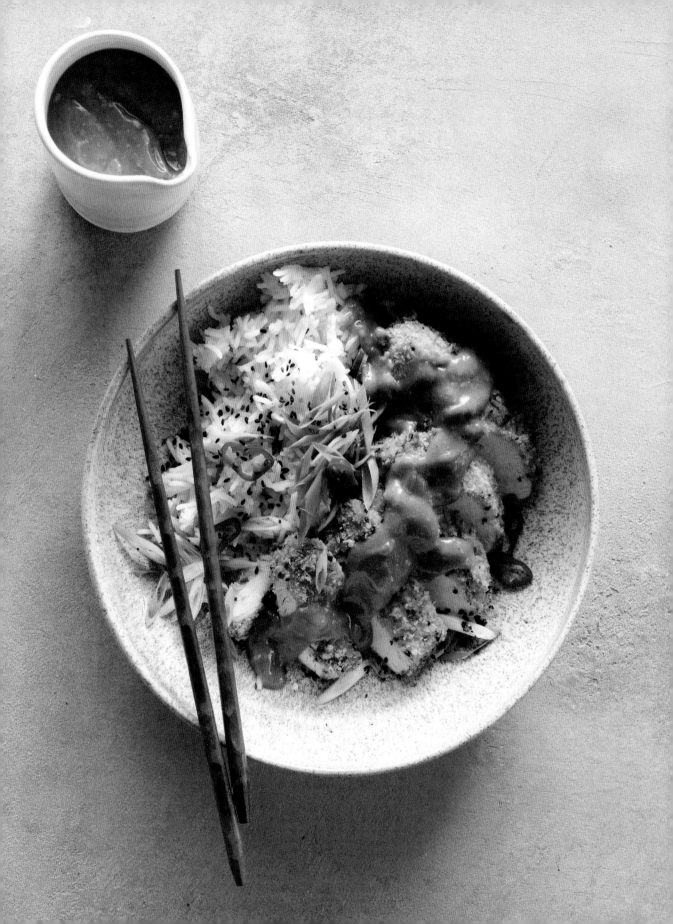

KATSU CURRY

Crispy chicken, curry sauce and rice, enough said!

SERVES 4

4 large chicken fillets

50g panko breadcrumbs

1 tbsp lemon pepper (you can use sea salt and black pepper as an alternative)

½ tsp ground ginger

1 tsp turmeric

1 tsp chilli flakes

1 tsp garlic powder

2 eggs

Low-calorie spray oil

700ml curry sauce of your choice

360g long-grain rice

1 fresh red chilli, sliced

2 scallions, chopped

Black sesame seeds (optional)

1 If not using an airfryer, preheat the oven to 220°C.

2 Okay, so you want to start with two bowls, one for the chicken coating and one for the beaten egg.

3 In the first bowl, put the panko breadcrumbs, lemon pepper, ginger, turmeric, chilli flakes and garlic powder and give it a good aul mix.

4 In the second bowl, beat your eggs.

5 Next, remove all the scaldy bits from the chicken fillets (you all know what I'm talking about).

6 Dip a fillet into the egg, shake a bit, then into the breadcrumbs, making sure it's completely coated. Repeat with the other three fillets.

7 I like to cook them in the airfryer with a spray of rapeseed oil for 20–25 minutes at 190°C, or you can pop on a baking tray and cook in the preheated oven for 25 minutes, turning halfway through.

8 While the chicken is cooking prepare your rice and curry sauce.

9 Once the chicken is cooked and is golden and crisp, slice into strips, serve on a bed of rice and pour over the curry sauce. Garnish with fresh chillies, scallions and a few sesame seeds just to be extra fancy.

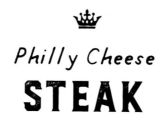

Philly Cheese
STEAK

The first cheese steak I ever had was in a small seaside town in Italy. The guy serving us was the owner and he talked us through the meat he used and where he bought his bread from a nearby bakery, then he unveiled a massive black pot that had the cheese sauce bubbling away. My mind was blown. I can still taste it now and it's something I've been making ever since.

SERVES 2-3

Low-calorie spray oil

1 green pepper, deseeded and sliced

1 red pepper, deseeded and sliced

1 onion, sliced

½ tsp smoked paprika

½ tsp garlic powder

2-3 pinches chilli flakes

2 leaner option beef medallions

3 light cheese singles

2-3 wholemeal rolls

1 Spray a pan with the oil and fry up the peppers and onion. I like to jazz them up so I add in smoked paprika, garlic powder and chilli flakes. Once they have softened leave to one side until the steak is ready.

2 On a separate hot pan spray some oil and fry the steak to your preference. I like mine rare, so if the steak is thick, I fry it on a high heat for 5 minutes on each side until nice and brown but pink inside. Leave it for longer if you prefer it well done.

3 Remove from the pan and let rest for 5 minutes to allow the juices to recirculate.

4 Put the light cheese singles in a pot with 50ml of water on a medium heat, stir and let them melt until you have a nice smooth cheese sauce.

5 Grab your roll and cut it open. Slice up the steak and pile into the roll along with the peppers and onion, then drizzle over the masso cheese sauce.

6 Simple, delicious and soooo satisfying.

Chicken and Leek
VOL-AU-VENTS

I was never able to spell this – probably googled the spelling about 765 times and still got it wrong. Anyway, if you like to be fancy and have guests over and want to impress them, these are your lads. Vol-au-vents are traditionally served in puff pastry cases but I'm using wholemeal wraps to make them a little lighter – don't worry, they will still knock the jocks off your guests!

SERVES 3

3 chicken fillets, chopped

2 tbsp cornflour

Low-calorie spray oil

3 garlic cloves, crushed

2 large leeks, well rinsed and chopped

350g mushrooms, chopped

600ml chicken stock

1 herb stock pot

150ml skimmed milk

15g Parmesan cheese, grated

3 wholemeal wraps

1 egg, beaten with a little water (egg wash)

1 First make the filling. Coat the chopped chicken in the cornflour – I usually pop them in a bag and give it a good shake, making sure to hold the end firmly.

2 Heat up a wok with 4–5 sprays of oil and brown the cornflour-coated chicken, then add in the garlic.

3 When the chicken and garlic is cooked add the leeks and mushrooms and cook for 8–10 minutes or until softened.

4 Pour in the chicken stock, then add the herb stock pot and the milk, give it a good stir and bring to the boil for 2–3 minutes. Reduce the heat, cover the pan with a lid and simmer for 15 minutes, then add in the Parmesan. Stir again and simmer for a further 20 minutes until the sauce has thickened and reduced.

5 Now it's time to assemble the 'vol-au-vents'. Lay out a wrap and spoon 4–5 tablespoons of the filling on one half, wet the edges and fold the wrap over the top of the filling until you have a semicircle. Press the edges together and pinch with a fork to create a seal. Brush over some of the egg wash, which will add shine, and give 2–3 sprays of oil. Repeat with the other two wraps.

6 I cook mine in the airfryer for 10 minutes at 180°C or until golden and crisp; you can also pop on a baking sheet and bake in the preheated oven for 15–20 minutes.

7 Once ready, cut each wrap in half and serve.

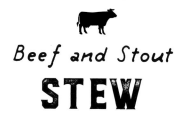

Beef and Stout
STEW

This is a massive family favourite and is proper comfort food for a cold winter's day. The kids lap this up so that's half the battle. A great way to get a bit of sneaky veg into their little bellies.

SERVES 4

1 kg baby potatoes, chopped in half

Low-calorie spray oil

2 tablespoons plain flour

Salt and pepper to taste

3 or 4 lean steak medallions, cut into chunks

1 large onion, finely diced

1 beef stock pot, mixed with 600ml boiling water

2 large carrots, sliced

150g frozen petits pois

1 tsp garlic granules

1 herb stock pot

1 tbsp sweetener

500ml Irish stout

Fresh or dried parsley for serving

1 Preheat the oven to 220°C.

2 Let's start with the spuds: I leave the skins on and just chop them in half, rinse them and pop them in the microwave for 15 minutes, shaking halfway through. Once they are slightly soft to touch, lay them on a baking tray, spray with the oil and pop in the preheated oven for 20–25 minutes until golden and crisp.

3 While the spuds are cooking you can get on with the stew. Put the flour in a mixing bowl, season with salt and pepper and toss in the beef chunks making sure each one is well coated.

4 Spray a high-sided pan with oil (I use my trusty wok) and get it nice and hot, tip in the coated beef and fry until brown, then throw in the onion and fry off until translucent.

5 Pour the hot beef stock into the pan with the beef and onions and stir well, scraping any flour off the bottom of the pan to mix with the liquid and thicken the sauce.

6 Add in your prepped carrots and petits pois, then add the garlic granules, the herb stock pot, the sweetener and then the best part – the stout! Mix everything together well and bring it to a boil.

7 Cover with a lid and leave it simmer for 1½ hours, stirring regularly so as not to let the meat stick to the bottom of the pan. The sauce will start to reduce and thicken and the beef will go so nice and tender. Give it a taste and add some salt and pepper if needed.

8 Serve in a bowl with your crispy roast potatoes on the side and a sprinkle of parsley. A deadly winter warmer!

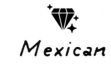

Mexican

CHILLI BOWL

This is perfect for a Friday night or Saturday night fakeaway, when you crave a junk dinner but don't want to give in to those cravings. Well, look no further, this will hit the spot. It's ideal for sharing and will fill up the hungriest of feasters. What's best is that it can be batch cooked and is also great to freeze.

SERVES 4

500 g lean minced beef

1 tsp dark soy sauce

1 large onion, finely chopped

1 red pepper, deseeded and sliced

400g passata

½ tsp garlic powder

½ tsp smoked paprika

½ tsp chilli powder

A pinch of chilli flakes (to taste)

1 tbsp sweetener

300 ml beef stock

3 large tomatoes, quartered

For the garnish:

Cheese sauce (see page 134)

Jalapeños (from a jar)

Homemade tortilla chips (see page 95)

1 Brown the mince with the soy sauce in a large wok, add in the onion and pepper and cook until they are softened.

2 Add in the passata, the spices and the sweetener and mix well.

3 Pour in the beef stock, throw in the fresh tomatoes, stir and cover with a lid. Simmer for 10 minutes until the sauce thickens.

4 Serve in a bowl drizzled with my epic cheese sauce, scattered jalapeños and some homemade tortilla chips on the side for scooping.

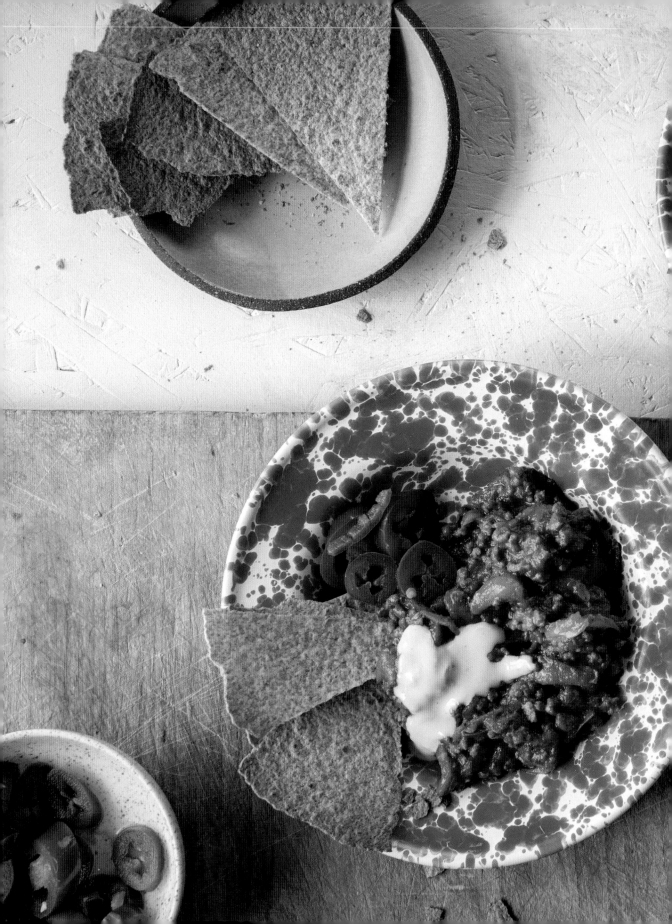

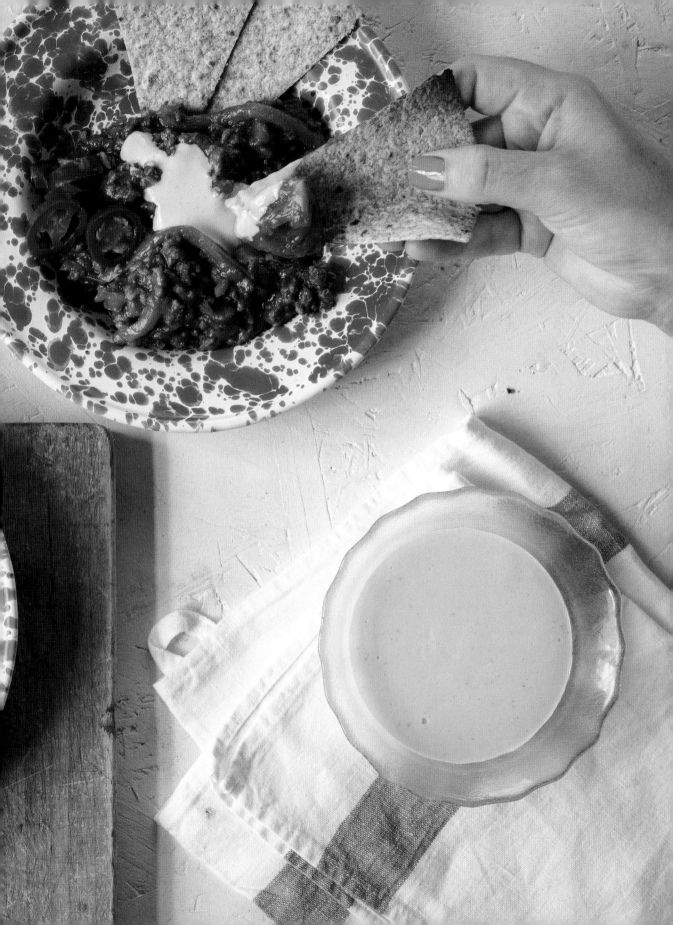

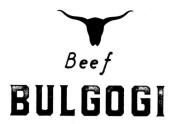

Beef

BULGOGI

Bulgogi, which translates as 'fire meat', is made of thin, marinated slices of beef or pork grilled on a griddle or pan. The dish originated from Korea and is one I always look out for when we are eating out. It's light and tasty and not full of nasties. Here is a version I cook at home and I know you will love it too.

SERVES 4

3 lean beef medallions

Low-calorie spray oil

For the marinade:

6 tbsp soy sauce

2 tbsp sweetener

2 tbsp rice wine

1 red apple, peeled, cored and finely grated

3 garlic cloves, minced

1 tsp ginger paste

½ tsp lemon pepper

2 tsp chilli flakes

1 tsp sesame oil

For the garnish:

2 scallions, chopped

1 tbsp toasted sesame seeds

1 fresh red chilli, sliced

Some lettuce leaves [optional]

1 Put all the marinade ingredients into a medium-sized bowl and mix well.

2 With a sharp knife cut up the beef into thin slices, add the bowl of marinade and mix well. Cover with cling film and pop in the fridge for 2–3 hours or overnight if possible to get the best flavour.

3 Spray a non-stick pan or skillet with some oil, heat it up, and add in the meat and marinade, stirring as it browns. The meat should cook superfast but you want it to be browned and charred, not steaming, so don't overload the pan. If need be you can do it in two batches.

4 Once the beef is cooked pour it onto a large serving plate and garnish with the scallions, sesame seeds and fresh chilli. If you want a bit of greenery, add some lettuce leaves to the mix.

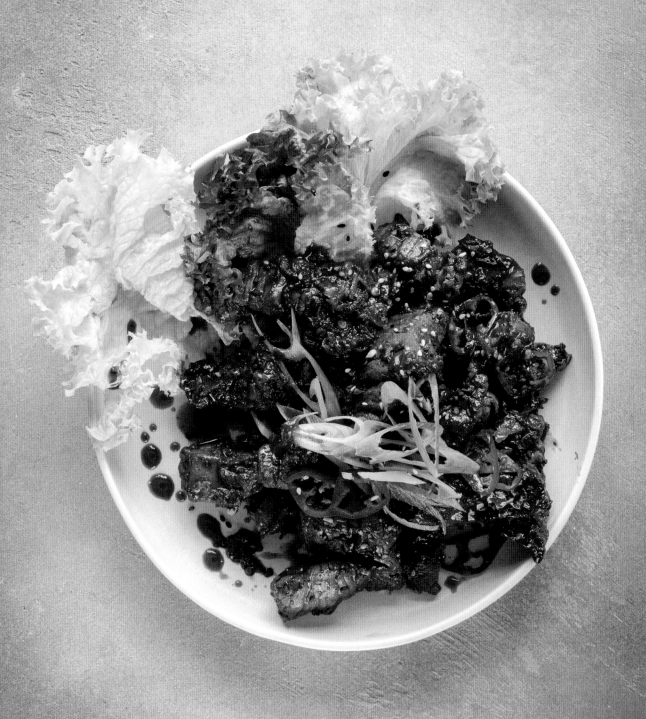

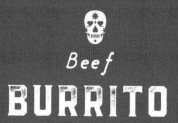

Beef

BURRITO

Mexican night is one of our favourite nights in my house. Even the kids love this little spicy number. Bang on the tunes and get cooking, this will be one you will repeat on the weekly!

SERVES 4

Low-calorie spray oil

500g lean minced beef

1 tsp soy sauce

1 tsp paprika

1 tsp smoked paprika

½ tsp chilli flakes

1 tsp garlic powder

½ tsp chilli powder

1 tbsp hot sauce

½ x 400g tin of red kidney beans, drained

1 red pepper, deseeded and sliced

1 onion, sliced

1 x 400g tin refried beans

200g cooked rice

1 small tin of sweetcorn, drained

4 wholemeal wraps

30g Cheddar cheese, grated

Light sour cream

1 Start by making the filling. Heat up a wok with 4–5 sprays of oil and brown the mince, then add in the soy sauce, paprika, smoked paprika, chilli flakes, garlic powder, chilli powder and hot sauce.

2 Add in the kidney beans, stir well, then add in 100ml of water to loosen the mixture and create a small bit of sauce.

3 In a separate pan fry off your pepper and onion until the onion is translucent and leave to one side.

4 Mix the rice (which must be recently cooked) with the sweetcorn and leave to one side.

5 Now it's time to assemble your burritos. Warm the wraps for about a minute in the microwave to soften. Now lay them out, add a layer of refried beans down the centre of each one, then dollop on the mince mixture, a few spoonfuls of rice and sweetcorn, some pepper and onions, a sprinkle of cheese and a few dollops of light sour cream.

5 Hold the sides of the wrap and give all the ingredients a little shake to mix together, wrap that bad boy up and repeat with the remainder of the wraps and mixture. This will be so bursting with flavour, you'll probably want a second one.

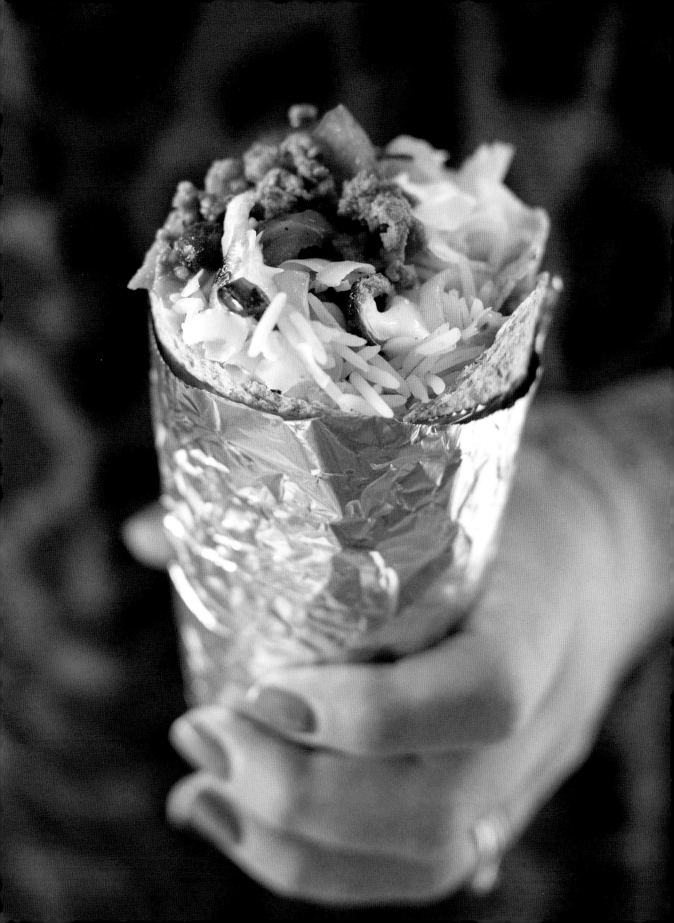

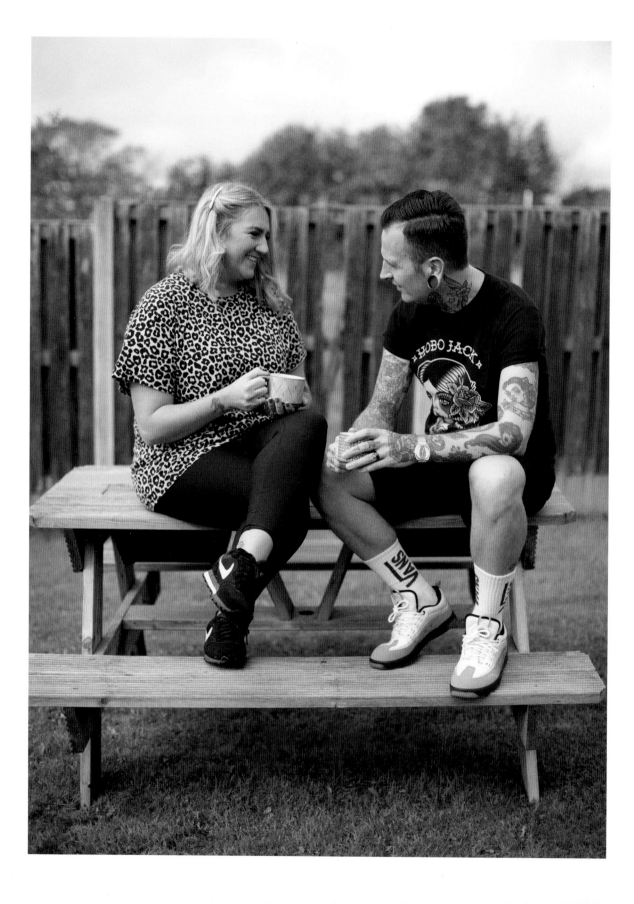

COTTAGE PIE

A tasty hearty family favourite that's perfect to batch cook and freeze. Great for the weeks you are short on time and want to stay on top of things but still want a hearty meal to come home to.

SERVES 4

700g potatoes

500g lean minced beef

1 tbsp dark soy sauce

1 onion, finely chopped

2 garlic cloves, crushed

1 x 340g jar of baby carrots, drained

4 tbsp frozen petits pois

500ml beef stock

½ herb stock pot

100ml passata

Salt and white pepper to taste

1 tsp cornflour (optional)

1 I start by prepping my spuds. Peel and chop into quarters and put in a large pan of boiling water. When they have softened, remove from the heat, add a pinch of salt and pepper and mash.

2 Preheat your oven to 200°C.

3 Now heat a large wok/pan on a medium heat and fry off the mince with the soy sauce until brown (tip: if you add a drop of water into the pan it will stop the mince clumping together).

4 Add in the onion and garlic and cook until the onion is translucent. Add in the carrots and petits pois and warm through, pour over the beef stock and passata and add the half stock pot. Season with the salt and white pepper.

5 Stir well and bring to a boil, turn down the heat and cover for 15 minutes until the sauce has thickened; if it needs a little help you can add in 1 tsp of cornflour mixed with water to help thicken.

6 Once the beef and sauce are cooked, transfer into a medium-sized Pyrex dish, layer on the mash over the top and spread evenly until it covers all the sauce. You can make the whole thing a bit fancy by running a fork prettily over the top.

7 Cook in the preheated oven for 25 minutes or until the mash starts to brown and crisp up.

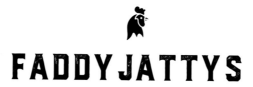

FADDY JATTYS

Also known as fajitas! This is a running joke; I heard it on a pronunciation video that was taking the mick out of loads of words and this one has just stuck. I don't think I'll ever be able to call them fajitas again.

SERVES 4

Low-calorie cooking spray

3 garlic cloves, crushed

4 chicken fillets, chopped

350 g chopped mushrooms

1 red pepper, deseeded and sliced

1 yellow pepper, deseeded and sliced

1 large white onion, sliced

1 fresh red chilli, sliced

4 wholemeal wraps

For the seasoning:

1 tsp smoked paprika

½ tsp chilli powder

1 tsp garlic powder

Salt to taste

For the garnish:

Light sour cream

Salsa (from a jar)

Fresh limes

1 Start by mixing all the spices for the seasoning together in a small bowl. Set aside.

2 Spray your wok with a little low-calorie spray and place on a medium heat. Add in the garlic and fry off for 1–2 minutes, then add the chicken and brown, keeping everything moving in the pan to cook evenly.

3 Add in the mushrooms, peppers, onion and chilli and cook until the onion is translucent, then sprinkle the seasoning mix over the cooked chicken and veg. You probably won't need it all – add it to taste.

4 Continue to cook for 2–3 minutes, adding 50ml of water just to loosen the spices up and coat everything evenly.

5 Toast your wraps on a hot dry pan for 1–2 minutes and spoon even amounts of the mix onto each one.

6 Garnish with some light sour cream and salsa and squeeze over some fresh lime juice.

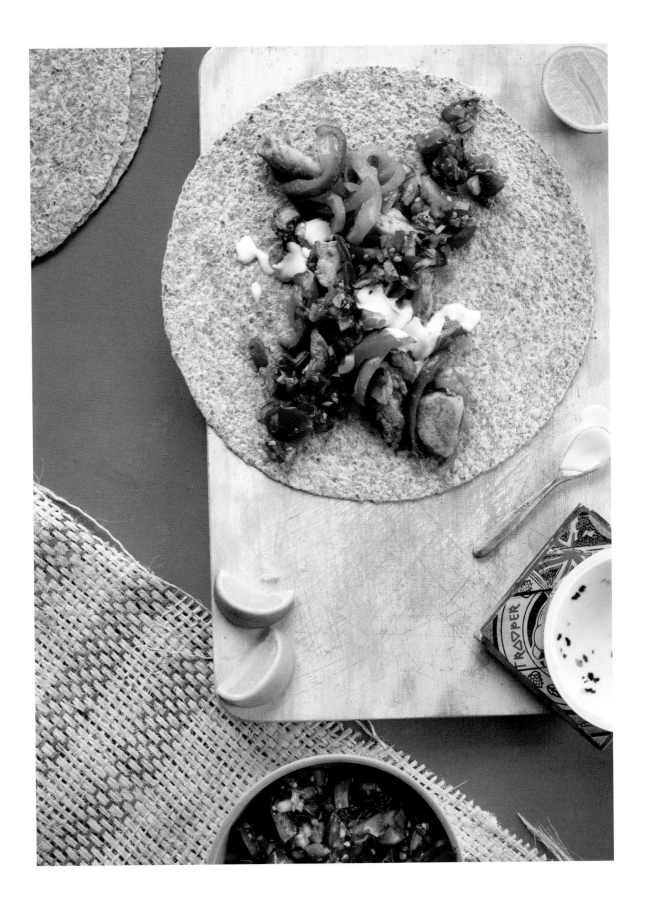

★★★
CHICKEN KIEV

My ultimate childhood favourite dinner was chicken Kiev – I probably had it about four times a week and I'm sure the kids in school hated sitting beside me, cause I'd be reeking of garlic! But that didn't stop me and I still love an aul Kiev to this day.

SERVES 4

4 large chicken fillets

50g instant mash (in its dry form)

2 tbsp lemon pepper (this is the secret ingredient)

½ tsp turmeric

2 eggs, whisked

Low-calorie spray oil

For the garlic butter:

4 garlic cloves, minced

4 level tbsp light butter

1 tsp dried parsley

1 To make the garlic butter, put all the ingredients into a small bowl and mash together with a fork. Lay out some cling film and spoon on the mixture. Roll it up into a fat sausage shape and pop into the freezer for 1 hour until it's firm.

2 Lay out the chicken fillets on some cling film/wrap and bash them with a meat tenderiser or a rolling pin until they are flat.

3 Grab the hardened butter from the freezer, slice into four equal pieces and pop one onto the middle of each chicken fillet.

4 Roll up the stuffed chicken pieces like burritos, tucking in the sides, wrap each one in fresh cling film and pop in the fridge for 1–2 hours to set.

5 When they are ready, remove the cling film. Preheat the oven to 180°C.

6 Mix the instant mashed potato with the lemon pepper and turmeric.

7 Dip each fillet into the whisked egg and then into the coating.

8 Lay out the Kievs on a baking tray and give each one 4–5 sprays of low-calorie spray oil.

4 Cook in the preheated oven for 20–25 minutes, turning halfway through and respraying until they are cooked through and golden brown and crisp all over.

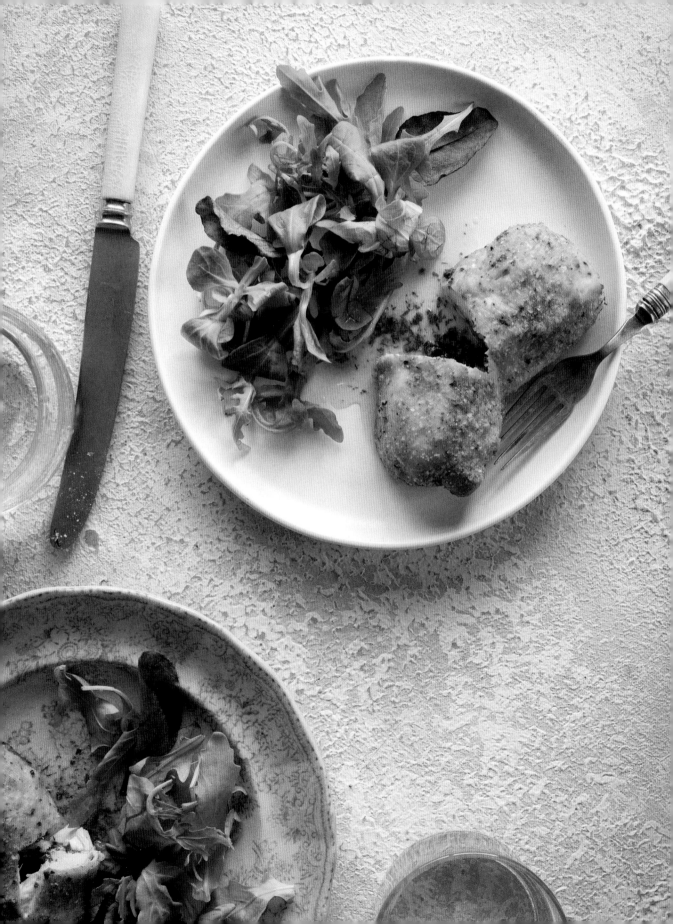

VEGAN BURGERS

Simple, tasty and handy AF to make. These work great as a burgers or, once cooked, can be kept in the fridge and cut up for salads or wraps. A great little nutritious snack and also great for the lunchbox.

SERVES 8

150g frozen cauliflower florets

1 x 400g tin of chickpeas, drained

100g carrots from a jar, drained

70g tinned sweetcorn, drained

40g porridge oats

2 tbsp buffalo hot sauce

1 tsp garlic granules

1 tsp smoked paprika

1 tsp onion granules

½ tsp ground ginger

White pepper to taste

Sea salt to taste

1 Throw the cauliflower into a pot of boiling water and let it cook for 3–4 minutes. Drain and set aside

2 Pop the chickpeas into a food blender together with the carrots and sweetcorn. Give everything a good blitz until everything is broken down but you still have a chunky texture.

3 Transfer into a mixing bowl, add in the rest of the ingredients and mix well.

4 Heat a pan with a 3–4 sprays of oil. Take palm-sized pieces of the mixture and flatten each into a burger shape.

5 Pop onto the hot pan, turn down the heat to medium and cook in batches of four, allowing to fry for 4–5 minutes on each side.

6 Continue to cook until golden brown. These are delicious served with some hummus and pickled red onion, available in jars. You could also make your own by marinating a finely sliced onion in 200ml red wine vinegar and 1 tbsp granulated sweetener, for about 30 minutes.

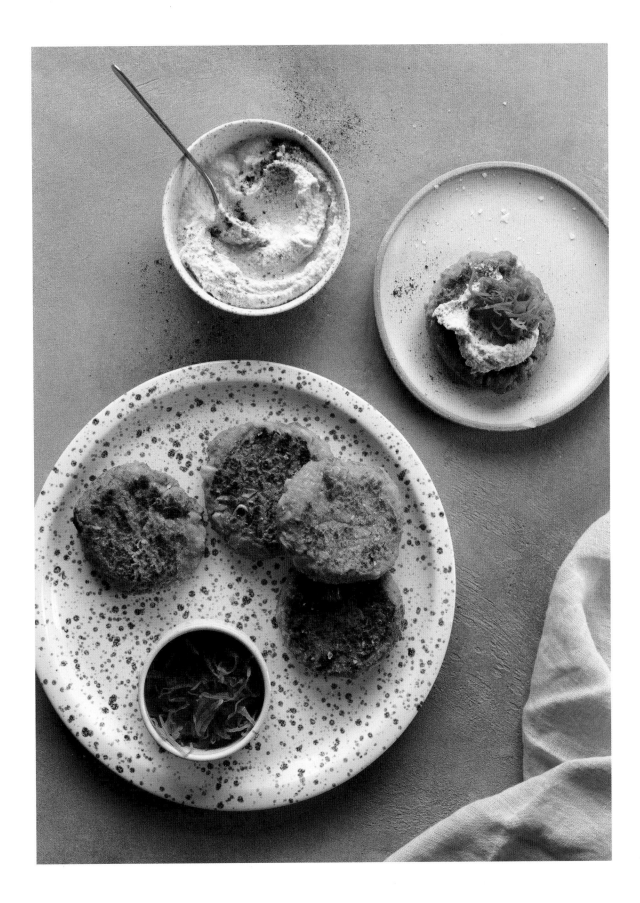

BUBBLE and SQUEAK

My favourite veg to have for a Sunday dinner are cabbage, sprouts and mash and we usually end with enough left over to feed the neighbours. This is a great way of using up all leftovers the next day. Easy, quick and super tasty.

SERVES UP TO 4

Low-calorie spray oil

4–5 smoked bacon medallions, chopped/leftover cooked ham/turkey

Leftover cabbage and sprouts

300g leftover mash

½ tsp garlic powder

½ tsp onion powder

Stuffing (not essential)

Salt and pepper to taste

Leftover gravy, reheated, to serve

Brown sauce, to serve

1 Heat a non-stick pan with some low-calorie spray oil and fry off the bacon, or alternatively add in the leftover meat.

2 Next throw in the leftover veg and stuffing if you have it, cook for 4–5 minutes until it starts to brown and heat through, then pile in the mashed potatoes and mush it all together.

3 Pat it down slightly and leave it to cook until the base starts to crisp and turn golden. Don't worry if the cabbage starts to make funny noises - that's why it's called 'bubble and squeak'!

4 Place a plate on top, flip the pan over then slide the bubble and squeak back into the pan to cook the other side.

5 Once it's ready, slice up and serve with some leftover gravy or a dollop of brown sauce.

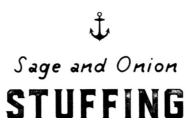

Sage and Onion
STUFFING

Nothing, and I mean nothing, could ever compare to my mammy's homemade stuffing. What I wouldn't give for it now! My sister Jackie, the little legend, perfected it over the years and it's something I always look forward to having. It's not just for a side with a roast dinner, this is fab loaded into a chicken sambo with some light mayo!

SERVES 3-4

Low-calorie cooking spray
½ small onion, finely diced
120g wholemeal bread
1 tsp dried sage
½ tsp mixed herbs
Salt to taste

1 Preheat the oven to 180°C.

2 Spray a pan with 2–3 sprays of the oil and place on a medium head. Add in the onion and cook until translucent.

3 Tear up the bread into a food blender, add in the herbs and give a good blitz until you a have a fine crumb.

4 Transfer to a mixing bowl and add in the cooked onion. Season with salt and pop into an ovenproof dish.

5 Spray the top with 4–5 sprays of oil and pop into the preheated oven for 15–20 minutes, stirring halfway through to ensure it's evenly cooked.

ASK
ME
AIRFRYER

PERFECT CHIPS

This simple and easy method will give you the crispiest and tastiest chips every time. I always get asked how I make my chips look so nice and, honestly, it's so easy – if I can do it, you can too!

SERVES 4

1kg potatoes

Low-calorie spray oil

1 Wash and peel your spuds and cut into chips. I like mine chunky but do them the way you like , whether it's wedges or skinnier French fries.

2 Pop them in a microwave-safe bowl and give them a good rinse under the tap, then drain ALL the water off; this is very important.

3 Pop them in the microwave and cook on full power for 12–13 minutes (less if making a smaller batch), giving them a good shake halfway through. You want them to be soft to the touch, but not mushy. Don't worry if they stick, this is just the starch; you can rinse them again in cold water after microwaving and this will unstick them.

4 At this point you can season with paprika or garlic granules, but I like mine plain and simple.

5 Next pop them into the airfryer at 200°C. It will take roughly 15–20 minutes to get them nice and golden, but pay attention to my special trick:

6 Every 5 minutes I open the basket and give the chips a little spray with my oil and a good shake. This ensures they all cook evenly and end up super crispy from the oil. If I'm cooking for a gang and I have to make a few batches, I leave the made ones in a bowl and just as my last batch is ready I throw them all back in together to heat them up (just make sure you don't keep eating them while you are waiting, 'cause, trust me, they are feckin' delicious!).

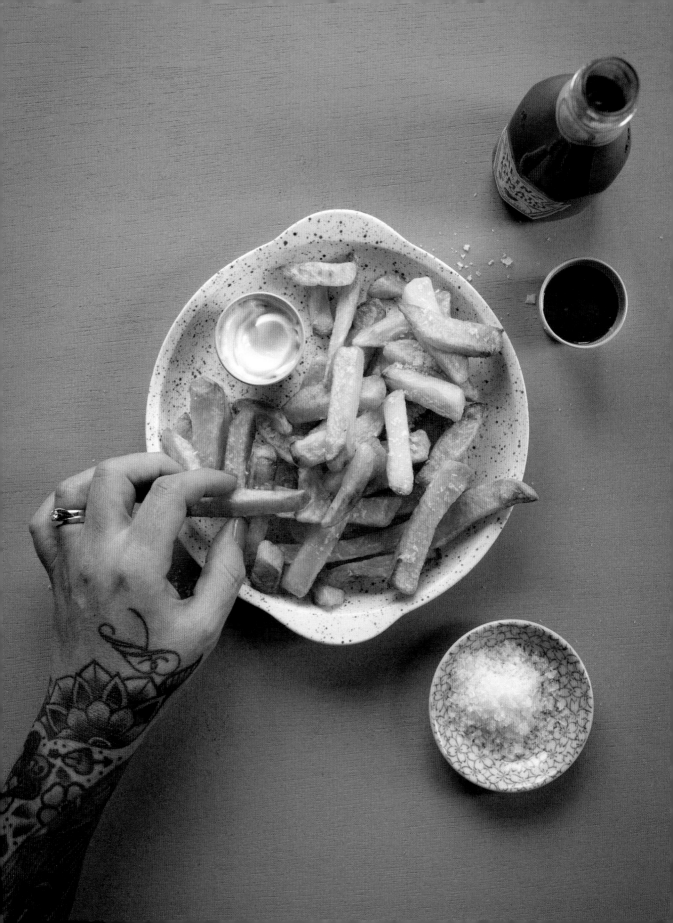

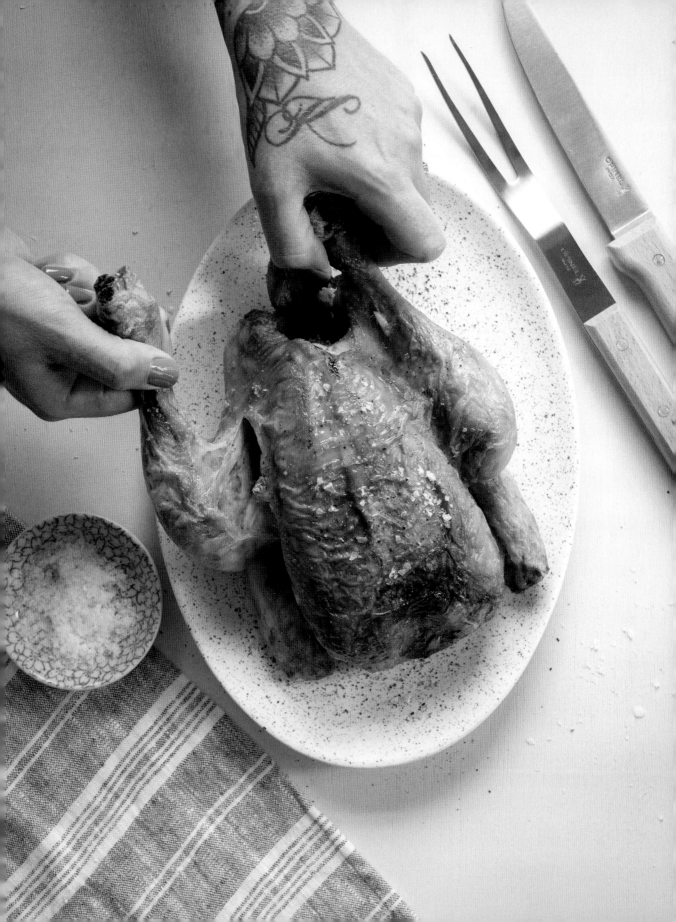

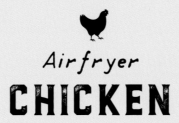

Airfryer CHICKEN

This is the only way I will cook my chicken now. It's quick, convenient and it doesn't make the whole house smell of chicken. You will get the most tender and crisp chicken with this method and will never look at your oven again! You'll need a large airfryer for this – mine is XL so it can fit a whole chicken inside.

SERVES 4

1.6kg whole fresh chicken
Low-calorie spray oil

1 I'm a simple gal and like chicken just as it is, but if you want you can season your chicken with herbs and spices of your choice, such as dried oregano or thyme, or some paprika.

2 Lightly spray the chicken with a small amount of spray oil and place it into the airfryer basket 'diddies down' (that's breast down to those of you not in the know). This will allow the juices to flow down into the breast rather than from the breast down and will give you a nice juicy bird.

3 Cook for at 180°C for 20–30 minutes per half kg, depending on the wattage of your airfryer. Flip the bird over for the last 20 minutes to crisp off the skin on top. When it's ready, remove from the basket and let it rest until you are ready to carve.

★ ★ ★

The Best Southern

FRIED CHICKEN

My first 'proper' job was working in a chipper! The wages were ridiculously low but the things I learned in those few years were priceless. They taught me how to make the best SFC ever. Now, while I know they deep-fried theirs, I have created a healthier version without the need for a deep-fat fryer that I guarantee will hit the spot.

SERVES 4

4 large chicken fillets

50g instant mash (in its dry form) or breadcrumbs

2 tbsp lemon pepper (this is the secret ingredient)

2 eggs

Low-calorie spray oil

1 If not using an airfryer, preheat the oven to 220°C.

2 Start by slicing your chicken breasts in half.

3 Put the instant mash powder (or breadcrumbs, if using) and lemon pepper into a bowl and mix well.

4 In another bowl, whisk the eggs.

5 Grab a piece of chicken and dip into the egg, then into the mash mixture and repeat until you have coated each piece fully.

6 Put the chicken in the airfryer with a spray of oil and cook for 20 minutes, turning halfway through.

7 If using an oven, lay the coated chicken pieces on a baking tray and spray with some oil, then pop in the preheated oven for 25–30 minutes until golden and crispy, turning halfway through.

8 Serve with fries and some gravy, or sandwiched in a burger bun with some lettuce, cheese and mayo.

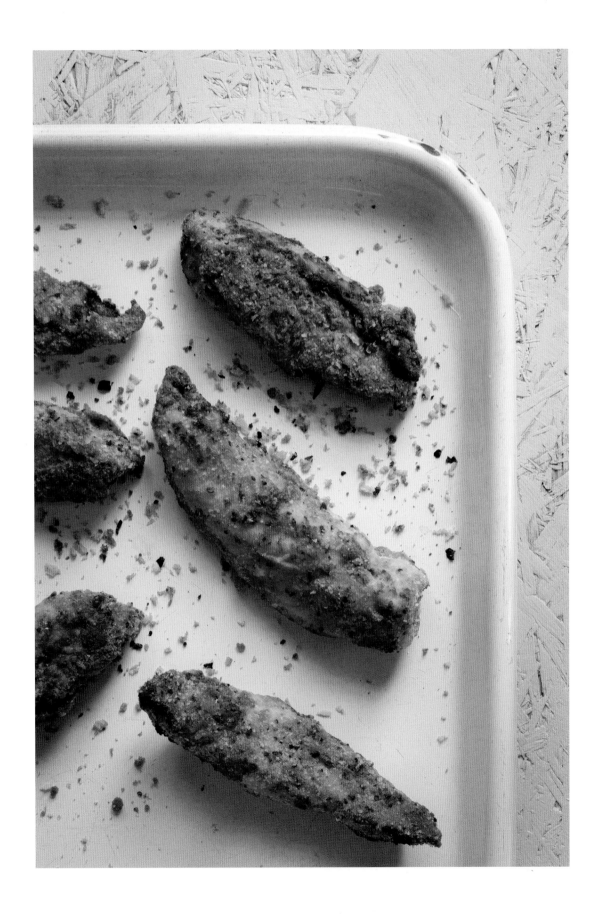

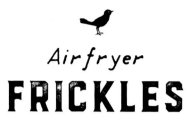

Airfryer FRICKLES

What the feck are frickles you say? Well, let me tell you! Frickles are fried pickles that are usually coated in flour and spice and then deep fried, but we're not going to do that. I have created a healthier version that is just as tasty.

SERVES 1

4–5 medium pickled gherkins

2 level tbsp cornflour

¼ tsp white pepper

½ tsp garlic powder

A pinch of chilli flakes (optional)

Salt to taste

Low-calorie spray oil

1 Slice the gherkins into ½cm coin shapes.

2 Mix the cornflour with the rest of the dry ingredients and dredge the sliced pickles in the mix until evenly coated.

3 Pop in the airfryer with 5–6 sprays of low-calorie spray oil at 180°C for 7–8 minutes, shaking halfway through, until golden and crisp.

4 Serve on their own as a tasty snack, piled onto a masso burger or as a side with chips.

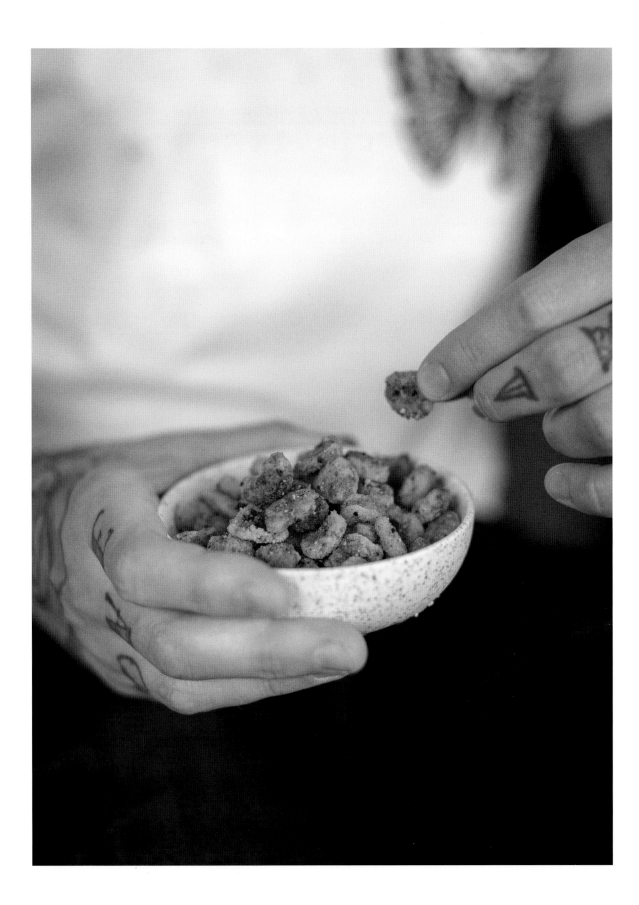

Honey and Sriracha-glazed Airfryer

BRUSSELS SPROUTS

Ehhhhh, no! I'm sure that's what most people think when they think of sprouts but when you jazz them up and airfry them they are actually masso. Trust me, just try them once!

SERVES 4

1kg fresh Brussels sprouts, trimmed and halved

2 tbsp honey

2 tbsp sriracha sauce

Salt to taste

1 Start by parboiling the sprouts for 3–4 minutes in boiling water to take the heavy bite out of them. Drain and pat dry and put in the airfryer for 15 minutes at 190°C.

2 Remove, pop into a bowl and add the honey, stirring well to ensure all the sprouts are well coated.

3 Pop them back into the airfryer for another 5–10 minutes until they start to brown.

4 Transfer into a serving bowl and drizzle over the sriracha sauce and a grind of salt to taste.

5 Serve as a side dish or on their own as a simple snack.

Veggie

FINGERS/NUGGETS

Not only will you love these veggie delights, they are a big hit with kids too. My little divils absolutely love these and it's a great way to sneak a little veg into their daily diets without them even realising.

MAKES 9 FINGERS OR 18 NUGGETS

250g potatoes, boiled and peeled

250g cooked carrots

4 tbsp frozen petits pois, cooked

4 tbsp tinned sweetcorn, drained

Salt to taste

Low-calorie spray oil

For the coating:

40g instant mash

1 tsp turmeric

¼ tsp white pepper

Salt to taste

1 If not using an airfryer, preheat the oven to 200°C.

2 Put the boiled potatoes and carrots into a mixing bowl and mash really well together.

3 Add in the peas and sweetcorn, season to taste with salt and mix well.

4 Spray some greaseproof paper with low-calorie spray and spoon out 2 tablespoons of the mixture.

5 With clean hands, shape into finger shapes, similar to fish fingers, or use half the amount and shape into nuggets.

6 To make the coating, mix the instant mash with the turmeric, white pepper and salt; the turmeric will give them a nice yellow colouring.

7 Sprinkle the coating over the fingers/nuggets, then turn over and repeat on the other side until they are evenly coated.

8 Spray with some low-calorie spray oil and pop them in the airfryer at 180°C for 15 minutes until golden and crisp. If using an oven, put them on a preheated baking tray and cook for 20 minutes, turning halfway through.

9 Serve with some homemade chips (see page 44) and a side of extra veg.

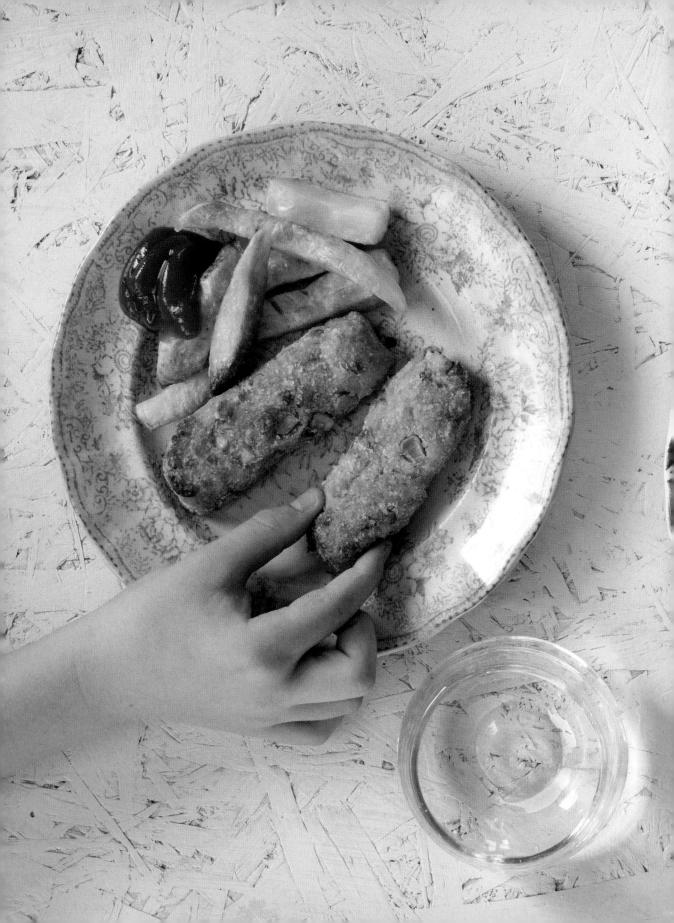

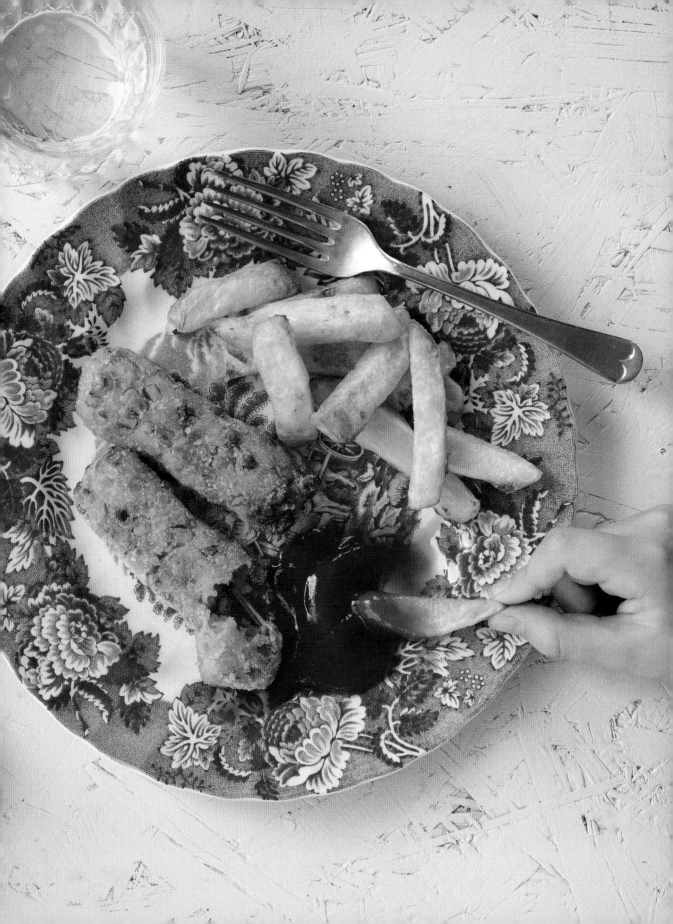

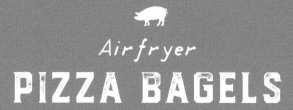

Airfryer

PIZZA BAGELS

The great thing about these little beauts is you can add any topping you want. They are quick, easy and so delicious. Nice for a little snack at lunch or served with some homemade fries for a satisfying dinner.

SERVES 1

1 wholemeal slim bagel, sliced in half

30g low-fat Cheddar cheese, grated

½ a pepperoni stick, sliced

1 tomato, thinly sliced

BBQ sauce (optional)

1 Arrange the tomato slices over each bagel half, then sprinkle over the Cheddar cheese.
2 Scatter the pepperoni slices evenly over each half and pop into the airfryer at 180°C for 5–6 minutes, after which time the cheese should have melted and the pepperoni should be nice and crisp.
3 Drizzle with a little BBQ sauce if you like.

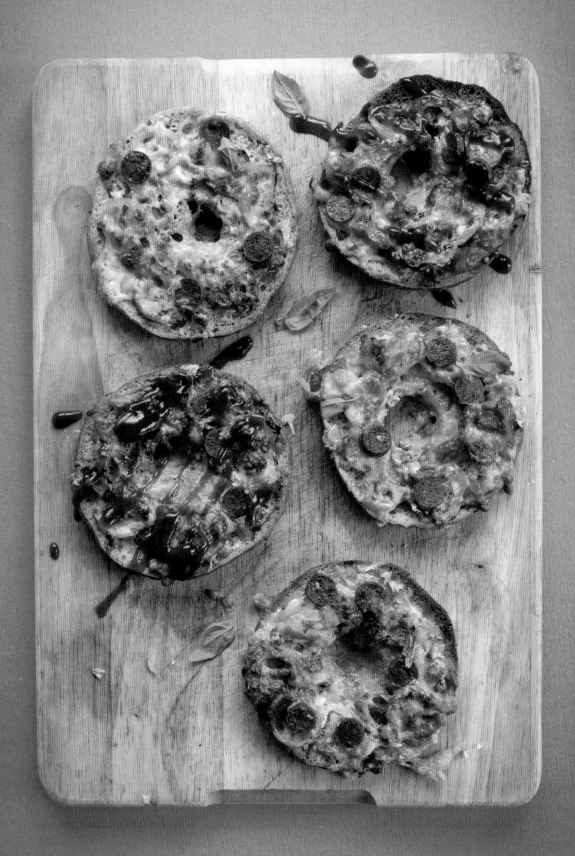

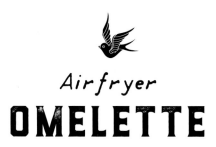

Airfryer

OMELETTE

This is a great way to get your omelette cooked evenly and to get the cheese in it to melt perfectly. Before embarking on the omelette, make sure your your airfryer has a flat bottom with no holes! This is a basic recipe just to get you started, but feel free to load it up with all the veggie goodness.

SERVES 1

7–8 mushrooms, cleaned and sliced

3 asparagus spears, chopped

Low-calorie spray oil

2 slices of ham, chopped

3 eggs

30g low-fat Cheddar cheese, grated

Fresh parsley, to serve (optional)

1 Pop the mushrooms and asparagus into the airfryer with a small spray of low-calorie oil and cook for 5–6 minutes until tender.

2 Add in the ham, then beat the eggs and pour these into the airfryer. Cook at 180°C for 6–7 minutes until your omelette starts to firm.

3 Open the airfryer, add in the cheese, then cook for another 6–7 minutes.

4 The cheese should be melted and golden and the omelette should be cooked through.

5 Grab a plastic fish slice, loosen the omelette all around the sides of the airfryer and slide out on to a plate. If you have some fresh parsley, sprinkle it over the top.

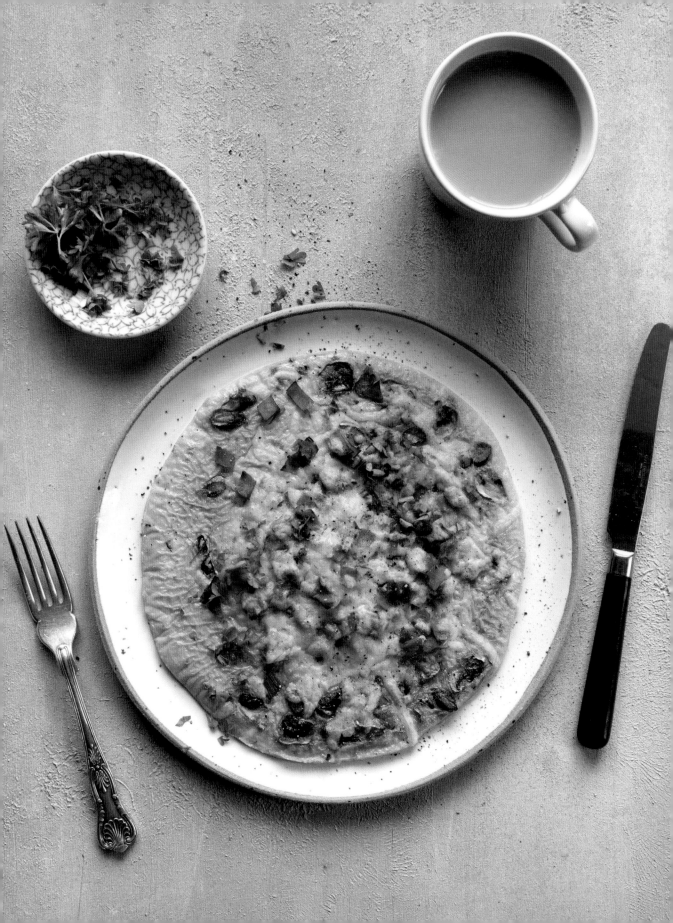

FAKE
MAKES

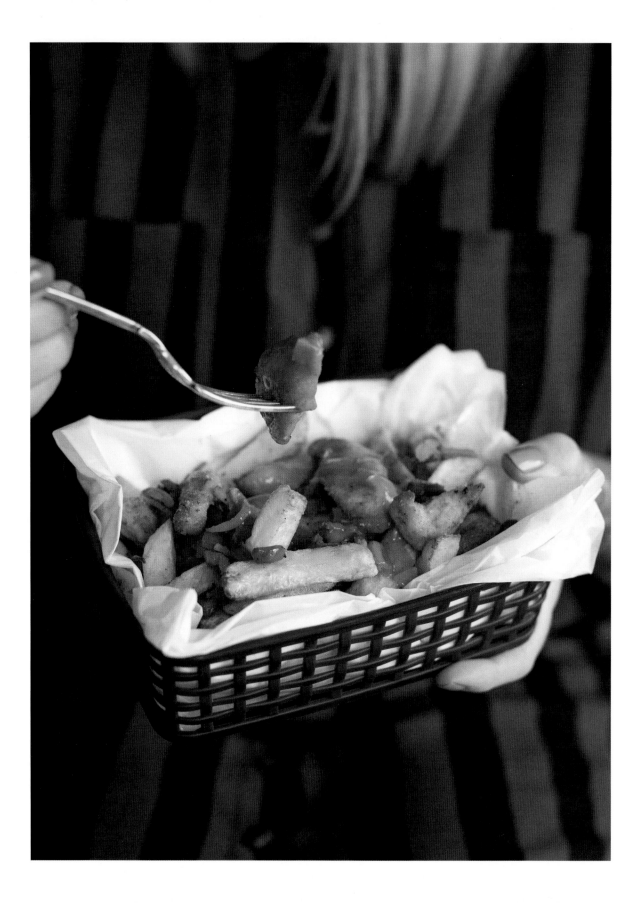

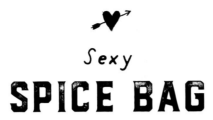

Sexy

SPICE BAG

A spice bag is actual life! They're so feckin' tasty and so easy to make! That's why I made it my mission to create a healthier version that would blow anyone's socks off. My version is packed with flavour and has all of that comforting goodness, but without the grease.

SERVES 2

For the crispy chicken:

40g instant mash (in its dry form) or breadcrumbs

½ tsp chilli flakes

1 tsp paprika

1 tsp garlic powder

Salt and freshly ground black pepper

2 chicken fillets, cut into strips

Low-calorie spray oil

For the veg:

3–4 large potatoes, peeled and cut into chips

1 large carrot, peeled and finely sliced into strips

1 large onion, sliced

1 red pepper, deseeded and chopped

1 garlic clove, minced

5–10 sprays of low-calorie spray oil

Salt to taste

Chilli flakes to taste

½ tsp Chinese five spice powder

1 tbsp sweetener (optional)

1 If not using an airfryer, preheat the oven to 200°C. First off we'll make the coating for the chicken. Get your instant mash and pour it into a medium-sized bowl. Then add all your spices and a pinch of salt and pepper and stir to combine.

2 Dunk and roll the chicken strips in the coating until they are nicely covered.

3 Throw them into the airfryer, give them a little spray with low-calorie spray oil and cook for 15 minutes at 180°C. Halfway through, give them a shake and a little respray of oil. When they are cooked, set aside to free up the airfryer.

4 If you don't have an airfryer, you can put the coated chicken strips on a baking tray, spray with some oil and pop them into the preheated oven for 20–25 minutes or until golden brown. Give them a turn and respray halfway through cooking.

5 Next up, rinse your chips and drain them well before popping them into a microwave-safe bowl and heating in the microwave for 8–10 minutes until they soften up.

6 Take them out, spray them with some oil and pop in the airfryer for 15 minutes at 200°C. Shake and respray halfway through cooking. Again, if you don't have an airfryer, just pop them on a baking tray, spray with oil and put in the oven with the chicken, until golden brown. Be sure to shake and turn them after 10 minutes.

7 When the chicken and chips are almost done, put the carrot, onion, pepper and garlic in a wok sprayed with some oil and cook until they have softened but still have a bite. Season as you cook with salt and chilli flakes to taste.

8 When the veg are ready, tip your cooked chicken and chips into the wok to warm them back up.

9 Add the Chinese five spice and sweetener, if using, and toss well to make sure everything is coated with the spices.

10 Then you're done! Dish up and serve. Drizzle some curry sauce on top, if you have it.

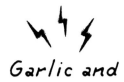

Garlic and

CHEESE FRIES

You'll never have to feel like you are missing out again with a takeaway essential that you can create right in the comfort of your own gaff! Oozy cheesy goodness.

SERVES 1

250g potatoes, peeled and cut into chips

5–6 sprays of low-calorie spray oil

1 garlic clove, crushed

3 tbsp lightest mayonnaise

A sprinkle of fresh parsley

3 light cheese singles, torn

50ml water

1 If not using an airfryer, preheat the oven to 220°C.

2 Rinse your chips and drain them well before popping them in a microwave-safe bowl and zapping in the microwave for 6–7 minutes until slightly soft.

3 Spray the chips with some oil, pop on a tray and put in the preheated oven for 15–20 minutes. If using an airfryer, pop them in for 15 minutes at 200°C, shaking and respraying halfway through.

4 In a small bowl, mix the garlic with the mayonnaise, sprinkle in the parsley and give it a good mix.

5 Put the cheese singles in a little pot with the water and stir over a medium heat until smooth.

6 When the chips are ready, put them in a bowl, smother with the mayo then drizzle over that masso cheese sauce. UNREAL.

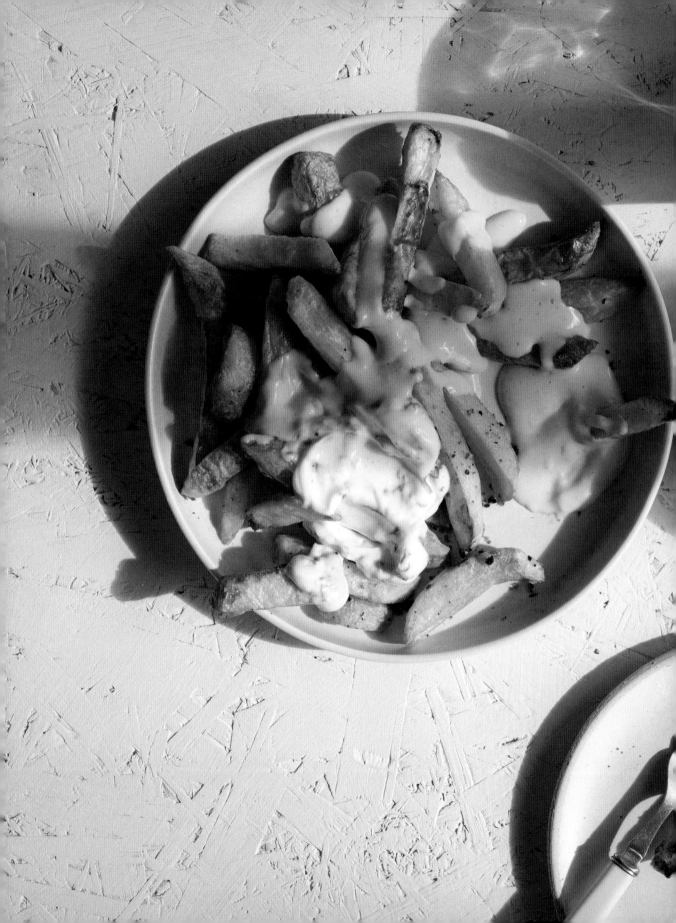

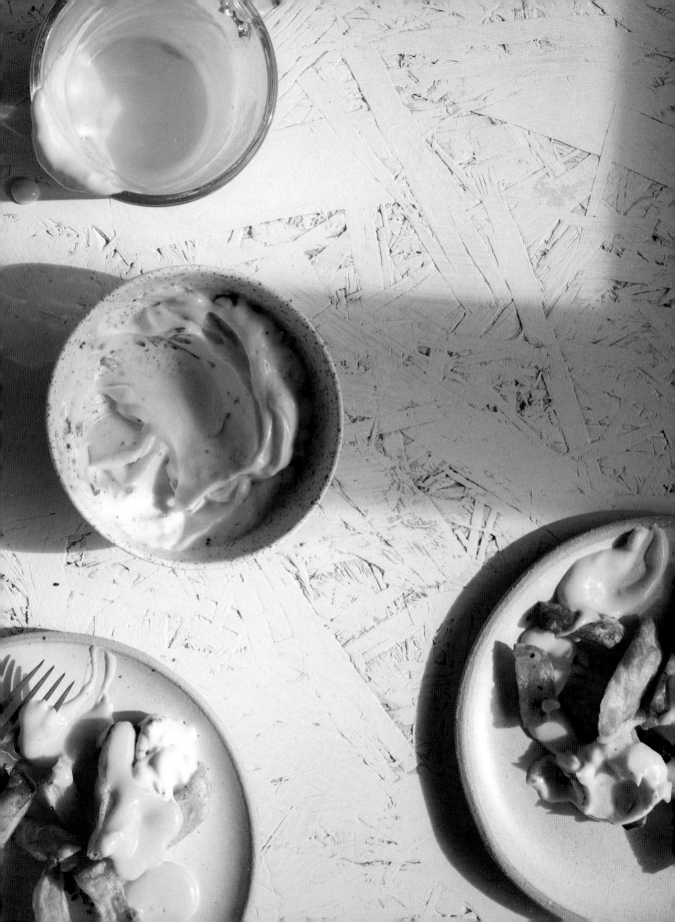

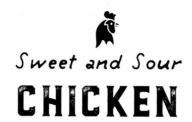

Sweet and Sour
CHICKEN

This will save you a trip to the takeaway and won't leave you with the takeaway bloat. Quick and easy to make and ideal for batch cooking.

SERVES 4

For the crispy chicken:

50g instant mash (in its dry form)

1 tbsp lemon pepper

4 large chicken fillets, chopped

Low-calorie spray oil

For the sauce and veg:

Low-calorie spray oil

1 green pepper, deseeded and chopped

1 yellow pepper, deseeded and chopped

2 garlic cloves, crushed

1 fresh red chilli, sliced

330ml zero-sugar orange soda

3 tsp soy sauce

1 tsp oyster sauce

2 tbsp passata

½ tsp ginger (fresh or ground)

½ tsp Worcestershire sauce

4 tsp white rice vinegar

½ tsp Chinese five spice powder

1 tsp cornflour

For the garnish:

A pinch of sesame seeds

1 spring onion, chopped

1 fresh red chilli, sliced

1 If not using an airfryer, preheat the oven to 220°C.

2 Mix the instant mash and lemon pepper together in a bowl, then add the chopped chicken and stir well until coated.

3 Lay out on a baking tray, spray lightly with the oil and cook for 15–20 minutes until golden and crisp, turning and respraying halfway through. If using an airfryer, pop them in for 15 minutes at 220°C, shaking and respraying halfway through.

3 Grab your wok, spray with some oil and place on a medium heat. Add the peppers and fry off, remove from the wok and set aside.

4 Spray the wok again and add in the garlic and chilli, allowing the garlic to brown for a minute or two.

5 Add in the orange soda and the rest of the ingredients (except the cornflour).

6 Bring everything to a boil for 2–3 minutes then bring down the heat and simmer to let the sauce thicken.

7 If the sauce needs to be thickened, mix the cornflour with 15ml water and add it into the sauce gradually until you have the consistency you want.

8 Toss in your crispy chicken and coat with the sauce. Serve sprinkled with a few sesame seeds and with the spring onion and chilli scattered over.

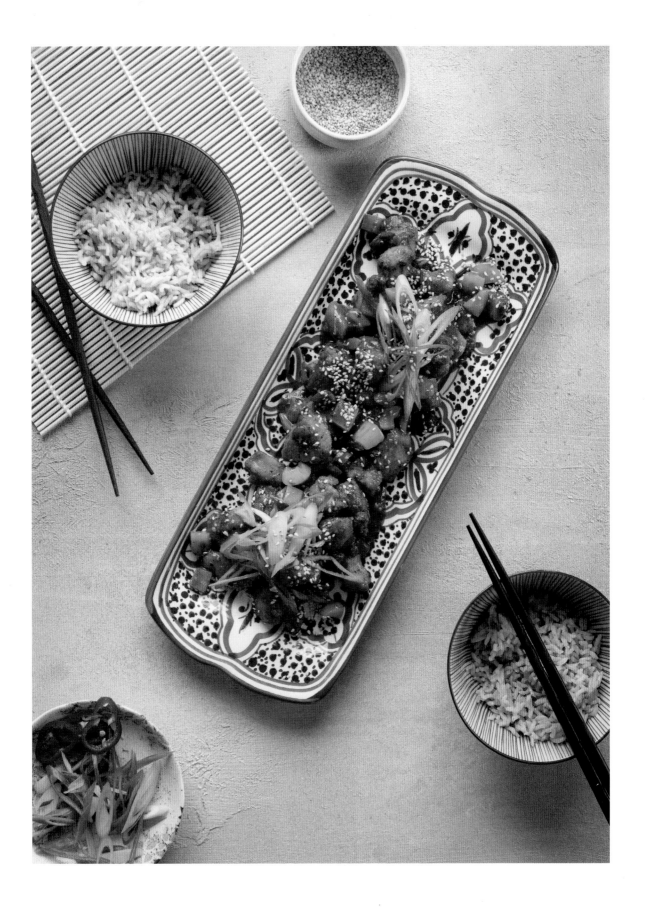

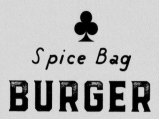

Spice Bag

BURGER

I love a spice bag and I love a burger, so it was only inevitable that this was going to happen: combining two of my favourite things to make one epic creation. This crispy chicken burger layered in a bun with veg and chips and drizzled with curry cheese sauce is just deadly!

SERVES 2

500g potatoes, peeled and cut into chips

Low-calorie spray oil

1 egg, beaten

25g instant mash (in its dry form) or breadcrumbs

1 tbsp lemon pepper

½ tsp ground ginger

½ tsp Chinese five spice powder

1 tsp chilli flakes

1 tsp garlic powder

2 large chicken fillets, sliced in half horizontally

2 garlic cloves, crushed

1 red pepper, deseeded and sliced

1 medium onion, roughly chopped

Salt to taste

3 light cheese singles, torn

50ml water

1 tbsp medium curry powder

60g wholemeal burger buns x 2

Iceberg lettuce, washed and torn

1 If not using an airfryer, preheat the oven to 220°C.

2 Start with the chips. Rinse and drain well before popping them in a microwave-safe bowl and zapping in the microwave for 12–13 minutes, then spray with the oil, pop on a tray and put in the preheated oven for 20 minutes. If using an airfryer, pop them in for 15 minutes at 190°C, shaking and respraying halfway through. When ready, leave to one side.

3 Put the beaten egg in a shallow bowl, then in another bowl mix the instant mash (or breadcrumbs, if using) with the lemon pepper, ginger, five spice, chilli flakes and garlic powder. Stir to combine. Now dredge your chicken pieces (which should be quite thin) in the beaten egg, followed by the spice mix, making sure each piece is coated evenly.

3 I like to cook the chicken pieces in the airfryer with a spray of oil for 20–25 minutes at 190°C, or you can put them on a tray in the preheated oven for 25 minutes, turning and respraying halfway through until golden and crisp.

4 While the chicken is cooking, prep your veg. Spray a little oil into a wok and add the garlic, fry until turning brown then add the pepper and onion. Cook until the onion is translucent and the pepper softened.

5 Now throw your chips into the wok with the veg, give a good twist of salt and toss them around for about 5 minutes to heat back up.

6 Meanwhile put the cheese singles in a small pot with the water and curry powder and stir over a medium heat until melted – this is going to be poured over the burger for extra massoness.

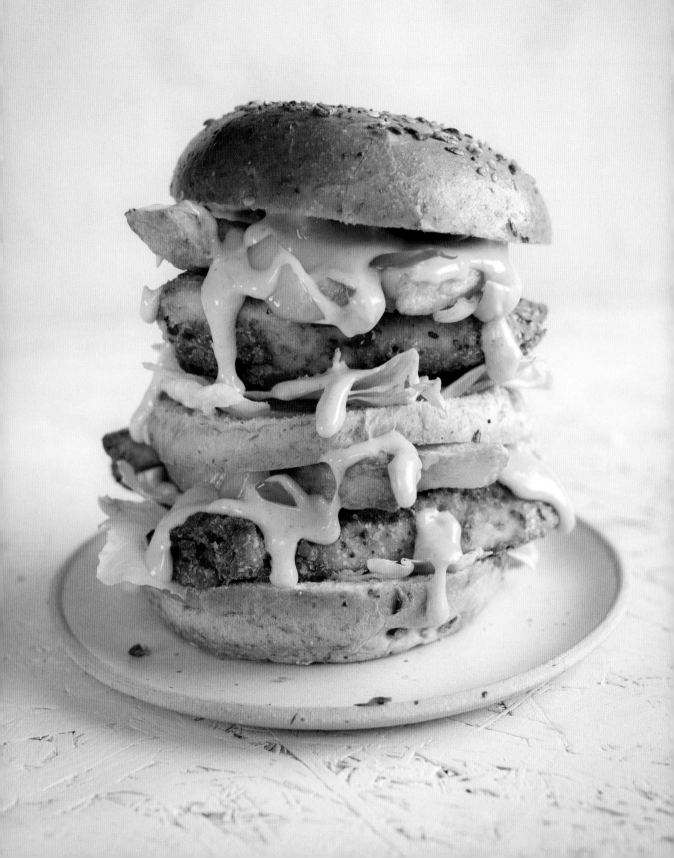

7 Now to layer this baby up.

8 Slice your bun horizontally into three (we are going to use one for the middle so that one can be thin enough).

9 On the bottom bun put some iceberg lettuce, one piece of the crispy chicken, some of the chips and veg mix, then pour on some curry cheese sauce. Pop on the middle bun then repeat the whole thing again until you have a sexy little tower burger. Repeat for the other burger and devour together in blissed-out silence.

Black Bean

CRISPY CHICKEN

This is probably the most-ordered dish from the takeaway for anyone on their 'night off' from a slimming plan. But let's be honest here, are you tempted to order it more than once in the week? Well I'm going to save you a trip and also a few bob. You can feed the family for the same cost as one portion from the takeaway and the best part is, it's all low in calories and so easy to make. Prepare to rock out with your wok out!

SERVES 4

For the chicken:

40g instant mash (in its dry form) or breadcrumbs

½ tsp smoked paprika

½ tsp chilli powder

A pinch of salt

4 large chicken breasts, cut into cubes

Low-calorie spray oil

For the sauce:

1 red pepper, deseeded and chopped

1 green pepper, deseeded and chopped

1 onion, chopped

2 garlic cloves, crushed

1 fresh red chilli, sliced

2 tbsp dark soy sauce

1 tsp oyster sauce (optional)

A 2cm piece of fresh ginger, grated

300ml chicken stock

1 tbsp black bean sauce (I use Lee Kum Kee brand)

1 tsp cornflour

½ tsp sesame seeds (to serve)

1 If not using an airfryer, preheat the oven to 220°C.

2 Put the instant mash (or breadcrumbs, if using), smoked paprika, chilli powder and salt into a bowl, toss in the chicken and stir to coat well.

3 Lay the coated chicken out on a baking tray, spray with oil and cook in the preheated oven for 20 minutes, turning and respraying halfway through. If using an airfryer, pop it in for 15 minutes at 200°C until golden and crisp.

4 Spray a little oil into a wok, place over a medium heat and fry the peppers and onion until softened, stirring regularly. Add in the garlic, chilli, soy sauce, oyster sauce (if using) and ginger and cook for a further 5 minutes.

5 Pour in the chicken stock and black bean sauce and stir through.

6 Mix the cornflour with a little water until you have a paste and add that into the wok, to thicken the sauce. Bring to a boil, then let it simmer for 6–7 minutes until you have a nice glossy sauce.

7 When the chicken is ready stir it into the sauce to coat fully. Serve with boiled rice and a sprinkle of sesame seeds.

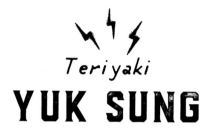

Teriyaki
YUK SUNG

I make up most of my recipes as I go along – I can taste what I want in my head and then just bring it to life. So it is with this gorgeous creation. Yuk sung is traditionally made with pork mince but I will be using beef in this recipe; you can also use turkey. Whatever floats your boat, Mary.

SERVES 4

500g lean beef mince

2 tbsp dark soy sauce

1 fresh red chilli, sliced

1 onion, finely sliced

2 garlic cloves, crushed

200g bean sprouts

½ chicken stock pot

150ml zero-sugar cola

1 tbsp teriyaki sauce

½ tsp chilli powder

½ tsp Chinese five spice powder

½ tsp ground ginger

8 iceberg lettuce leaves

1 In a medium-sized saucepan, brown your beef with the soy sauce, fresh chilli, onion and crushed garlic.

2 Add in the bean sprouts, chicken stock pot and zero-sugar cola. Stir well, then add the teriyaki sauce and mix everything together like a mad thing.

3 Add in the chilli powder, five spice and ginger and let it all cook for 5 minutes on a medium heat until the sauce thickens.

4 Once ready, spoon some into a lettuce leaf, fold over and enjoy this little gift to your taste buds.

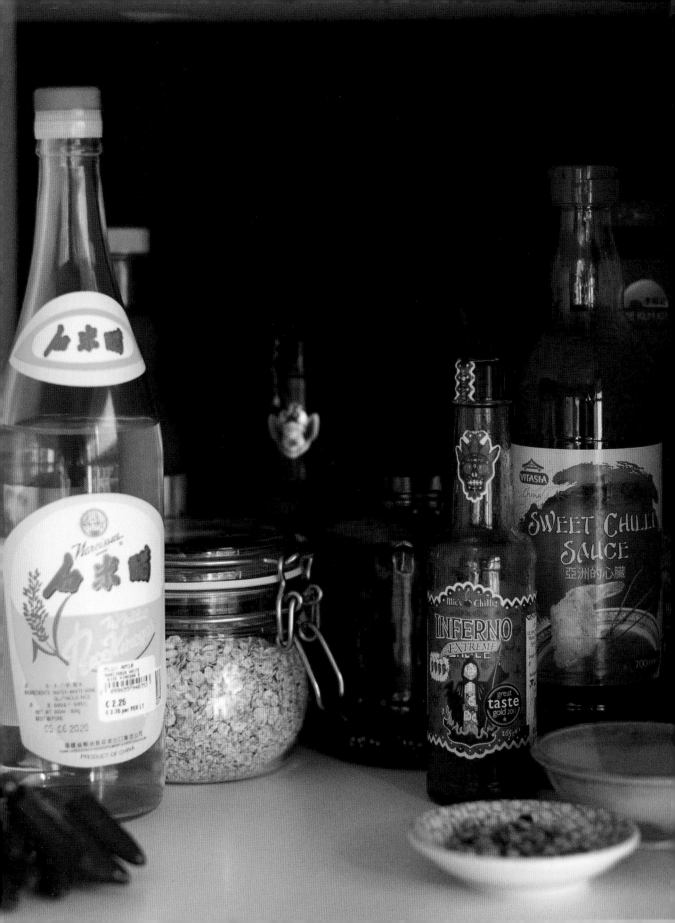

Super-speedy
SPRING ROLLS

I feckin' love an aul spring roll, but I bleedin' hate the grease dripping down onto my fingers, also the bloat and the guilt, so ... I made a Daly Dish alternative that is much lower in calories. I used rice paper and loaded them with vermicelli rice noodles and a rake of veg. Don't be put off by the lengthy instructions – I just want to make this recipe foolproof for you!

SERVES 2

4 asparagus tips

1 red pepper, deseeded and finely sliced

4 spring onions, finely sliced lengthways

1 carrot, peeled and finely grated

1 garlic clove, crushed

1 tbsp soy sauce

1 tsp oyster sauce

½ tsp Chinese five spice powder

½ tsp puréed ginger

1 block of vermicelli rice noodles

4 sheets of rice paper (you will find this in any Asian food market)

Low-calorie cooking spray

1 Get a non-stick pan nice and hot, throw in the asparagus tips, pepper, spring onion, carrot and garlic and fry off until al dente then add in the sauces and spices (but not the noodles yet).

2 Toss everything together and add a drop of water just to stop everything from sticking and to get a little sauce going that will coat all the veg.

3 For the noodles, put a block in a bowl, pour boiling water over it and let sit for 5 minutes, then drain the noodles and add them to the veg in the pan and mix well. Keep at a gentle simmer on a low heat.

4 Now for the rice paper. The stuff is very sticky, so keep your hands wet when handling. You have to wet it with warm water to get it to soften up and this is where you will either become a black belt in the art of spring roll making or you'll fire it out the window!

- Fill a large bowl with warm water.
- Take a rice paper disc and hold it between finger and thumb with both hands at the top.
- Dip it into the water and start to spin it quickly through your fingers in the water. Think of turning a car's steering wheel, with your fingers always staying at ten to two. The trick is to not let it soak, you are just giving it a quick spin in the water to dampen it all over!
- Lay it out on a piece of baking paper. Don't worry if it still feels a bit stiff, it will quickly go super soft and transparent and sticky AF (top tip, keep a little bowl of warm water to dip your fingers in for when you are ready to roll it up).

Okay ... hard part done, you then just want to add in the filling. Imagine the rice paper as a clock so I can tell you how to fold it:

- 🕐 12 o'clock is pointing away from you.
- 🕐 6 o'clock is pointing towards you.
- 🕐 3 o'clock is the right side.
- 🕐 9 o'clock is the left side.

5 Place a good portion of the noodles and veg in the centre of a prepared rice paper sheet and spread out.

6 Leave about 2 inches each side (left and right) and fold these towards the centre.

7 Then lift the 6 o'clock flap and bring it over the top of the filling and the tucked bits ... stick it down just behind the filling (kind of tuck it) and start to roll it until it's all nice and tidy and stuck together and looking like a spring roll, and that is the end of that! Thank fuck says you! Repeat the process with the other three.

8 You can eat them straight away or if you prefer them with a little crunch, pop them in the airfryer at 180°C for 10–15 minutes with a light spray of low-calorie cooking oil and they will crisp up!

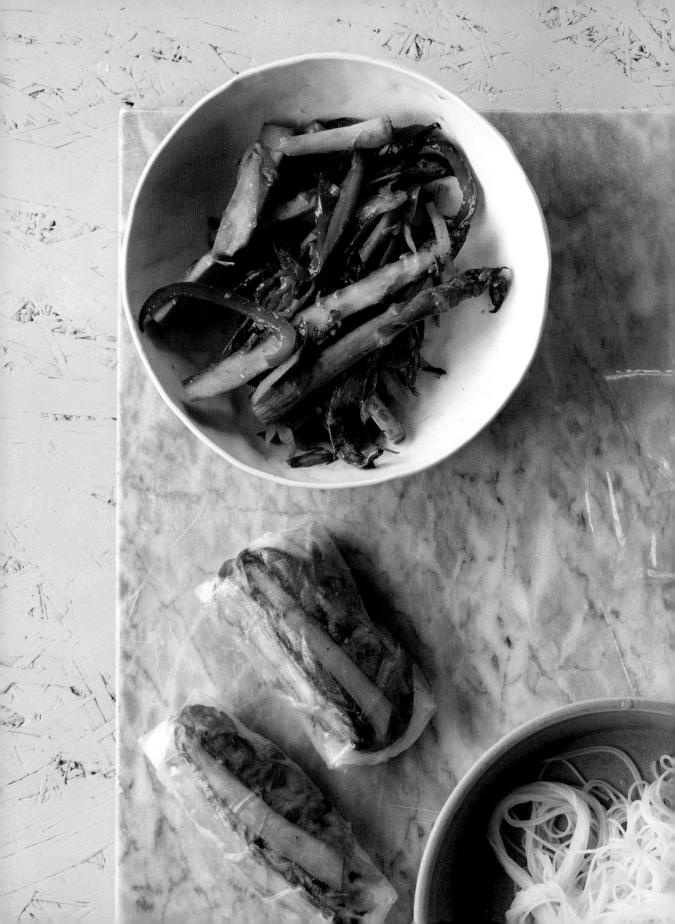

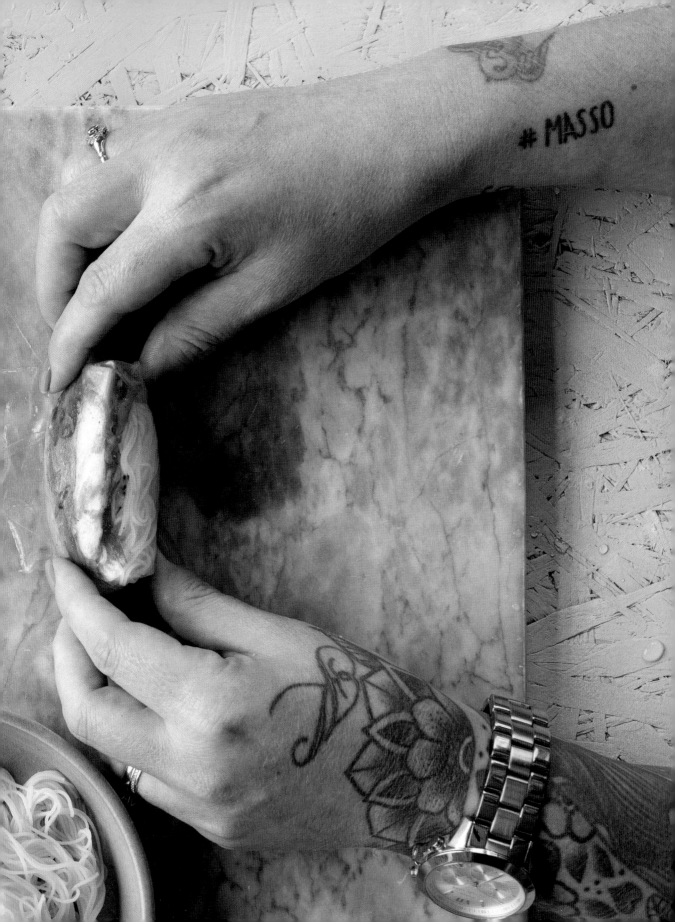

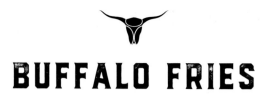

BUFFALO FRIES

Need I say more? The title says it all! These are incredible and are perfect for a night when you fancy a takeout-style dinner or some real comfort food.

SERVES 2

40g instant mash (in its dry form) or breadcrumbs

1 tsp smoked paprika

1 tsp garlic granules

A pinch of salt

2 chicken fillets, chopped

Low-calorie spray oil

4 large potatoes (for chips)

40g Cheddar cheese, grated

2 tbsp buffalo hot sauce

1 tbsp shop-bought Caesar dressing

Blue cheese (use as much or as little as your taste buds like)

1 If not using an airfryer, preheat the oven to 200°C. In a medium-sized bowl, mix the instant mash (or breadcrumbs, if using) with the paprika, garlic granules and salt. Toss the chicken pieces through to coat well.

2 Lay out on a baking tray and lightly spray with spray oil. Cook in the preheated oven for 20 minutes, turning and respraying halfway through. Alternatively add to the airfryer for 15–20 mins at 200°C, respraying and shaking every 5–6 minutes.

3 For the chips, rinse and drain, pop into a microwaveable bowl and zap in the microwave for 8–10 minutes just to soften up. Pop in the airfryer/oven for 20 minutes at 200°C, shaking and respraying every 5–6 minutes until golden and crispy.

4 When the chicken and chips are ready, build your fries! First place the chips on some baking paper and add a sprinkle of Cheddar. Toss the chicken in some buffalo hot sauce until coated entirely and add to the chips. Drizzle some hot sauce and Caesar dressing on top.

5 Then crumble over some blue cheese and add this back into the airfryer or oven for a few minutes until the cheese has melted.

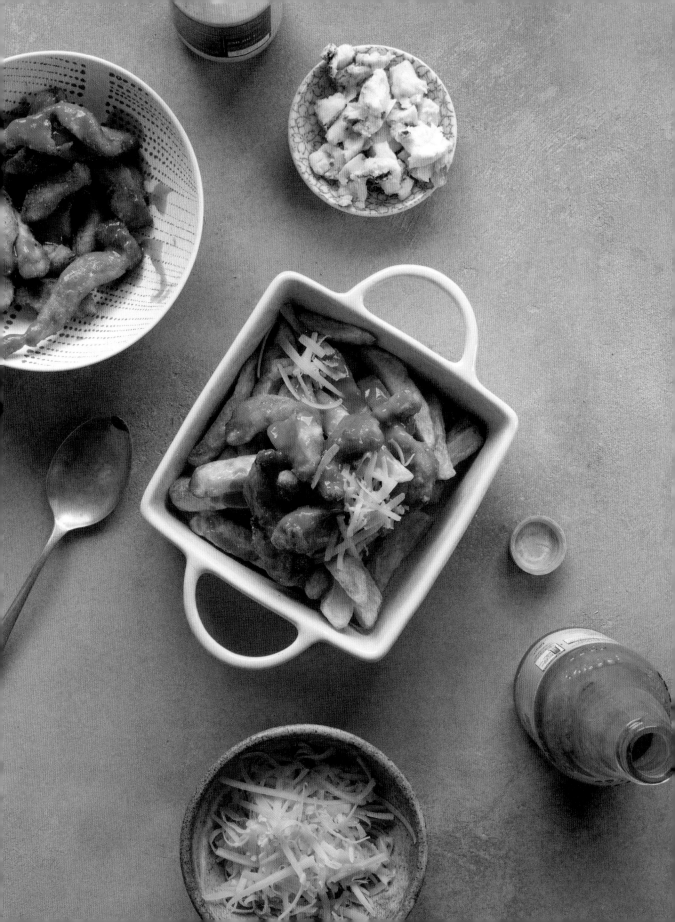

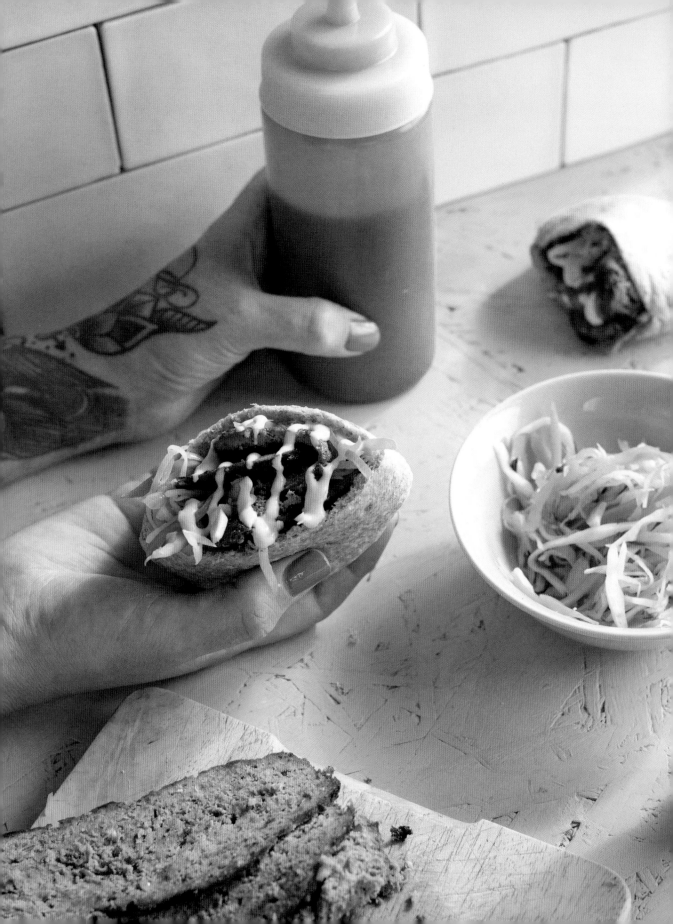

♛
DONER KEBAB

A traditional doner kebab is made with seasoned meat cooked rotisserie-style and then very thinly sliced. And I'm going to show you how to bring this takeaway classic to your kitchen without any fuss. We make this at least once a week and always have lots of leftovers we keep in the fridge to pop into a salad or to have stuffed into some warm pitta.

SERVES 4-6

1 onion, finely chopped

5 garlic cloves, crushed

Low-calorie spray oil

500g lean minced beef

1 tsp chilli flakes (if you want it spicy)

1 tsp cumin

1 tsp smoked paprika

1 tsp mixed herbs

1 tsp sage

1 tsp ground ginger

For the veg:

Low-calorie spray oil

1 carrot, peeled and grated

¼ white cabbage, shredded

1 onion, finely sliced

Salt and black pepper to taste

To assemble:

4-6 wholemeal pitta breads (one per person)

6 tsp shop-bought garlic sauce

6 tsp shop-bought chilli sauce

1 If not using an airfryer, preheat the oven to 200°C.

2 In a non-stick pan sprayed with a little oil, fry off the onion and garlic until softened. Transfer to a mixing bowl.

3 Add the mince and all the spices and herbs and stir together to let all the flavours mix well. You can get in there with clean hands and give it a good aul blend.

4 Empty out onto some greaseproof paper and tightly roll the mixture into a large sausage shape, then remove the greaseproof paper.

5 Pop into the airfryer for 25 minutes at 190°C or wrap in foil and pop into the preheated the oven for 35–40 minutes, removing the foil for the last 15 minutes to allow the meat to brown.

6 Remove and leave to rest while you get on with the veg. Put the carrot, cabbage and onion in a hot pan with a spray of oil and fry off for 3–4 minutes to take the crunch out. Season with salt and black pepper.

7 Heat up your pittas, slice the kebab meat nice and thinly, stuff into the pittas with the veg and drizzle over your favourite garlic and chilli sauce.

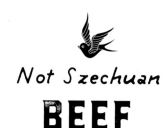

Not Szechuan
BEEF

Okay, so technically speaking this isn't Szechuan, because it's just not, but let's just pretend it is because it's just as feckin' nice. Szechuan beef uses Szechuan peppercorns, but I'm all about convenience and bringing you dishes with easily sourced ingredients so I have made a few tweaks and created something every bit as tasty.

SERVES 2-3

Low-calorie spray oil

1 garlic clove, crushed

1 fresh red chilli, sliced

1 onion, sliced

1 red pepper, deseeded and chopped

1 yellow pepper, deseeded and chopped

1 tbsp soy sauce

330ml zero-sugar lemon and lime

1 tbsp white rice vinegar

1 tsp ginger purée (available in jars)

½ tsp Chinese five spice powder

1 tbsp sweet chilli sauce

50ml passata

2 tbsp curry powder

2 lean steak medallions

Pinch of sesame seeds

1 Spray your wok with some oil and add the garlic and chilli, fry off for 2–3 minutes then add in the onion and peppers and cook for a further 5 minutes.

2 Throw in the rest of the ingredients (apart from the steak and sesame seeds) and stir well. Bring up the heat until it comes to a boil, then reduce the heat and allow to simmer for 10 minutes until the sauce reduces and thickens.

3 While the sauce is simmering, heat up a non-stick pan with some oil and throw in the steak medallions. How long you cook them for depends on your taste – I fry mine for 5 minutes each side for medium rare, but leave longer if you prefer them well done.

4 Remove from the pan and let rest on a plate nearby until the sauce is ready, then slice thinly.

5 Divide the sauce between two or three bowls, arrange the beef on top, then finish off with a sprinkle of sesame seeds.

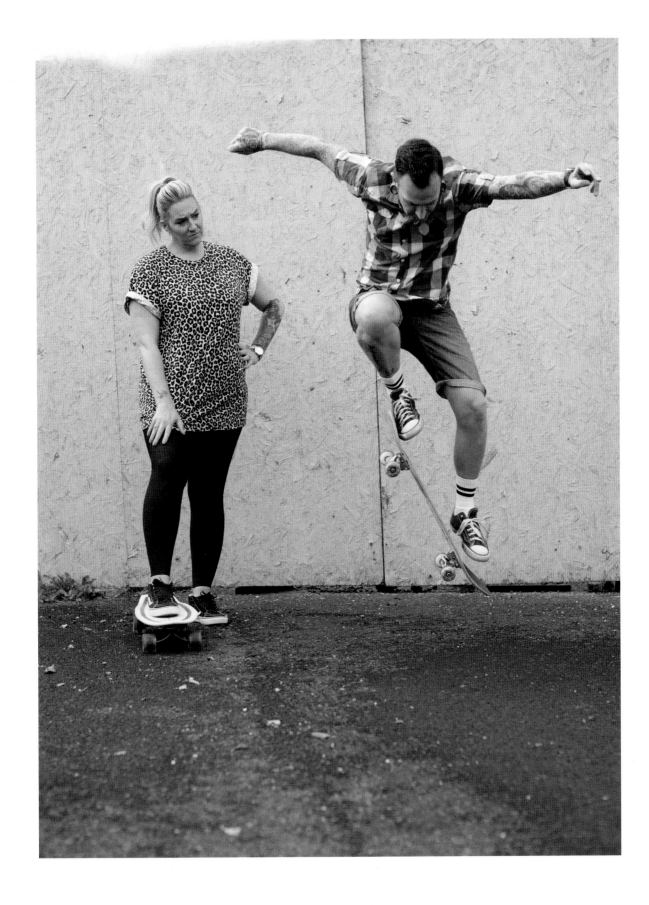

Chicken

FRIED RICE

Quick and easy and ready in less that 15 minutes, this is perfect as a meal on its own. You can bulk it up with any extra veg you have to hand – just add them when you're sautéing the onions and peas.

SERVES 4

Low-calorie spray oil

4 spring onions, sliced

60g frozen petits pois

2 x 280g packs of cooked basmati rice

3 chicken breasts, cooked and shredded

4 tbsp soy sauce

Salt to taste

White pepper to taste

2 large eggs, beaten

1 Spray a large wok with some oil and place over a medium heat. Pop in the spring onions and petits pois and cook for 2–3 minutes.

2 Add in the rice direct from the pack so it's cold going into the pan, mix with the veg then add in the shredded chicken. Throw in the soy sauce and toss everything in the pan for 2–3 minutes until the rice is warmed through. Season with the salt and pepper.

3 Make a big circle (about the size of your palm) in the centre of the rice and pour the beaten egg into it. Leave for 30 seconds or so until it starts to cook.

4 Using a spatula give the egg a good mix in the centre until it starts to resemble a broken-up omelette, then work it in to the rice, making sure it's evenly distributed throughout.

5 Continue to toss or stir for 2–3 minutes and serve in bowls.

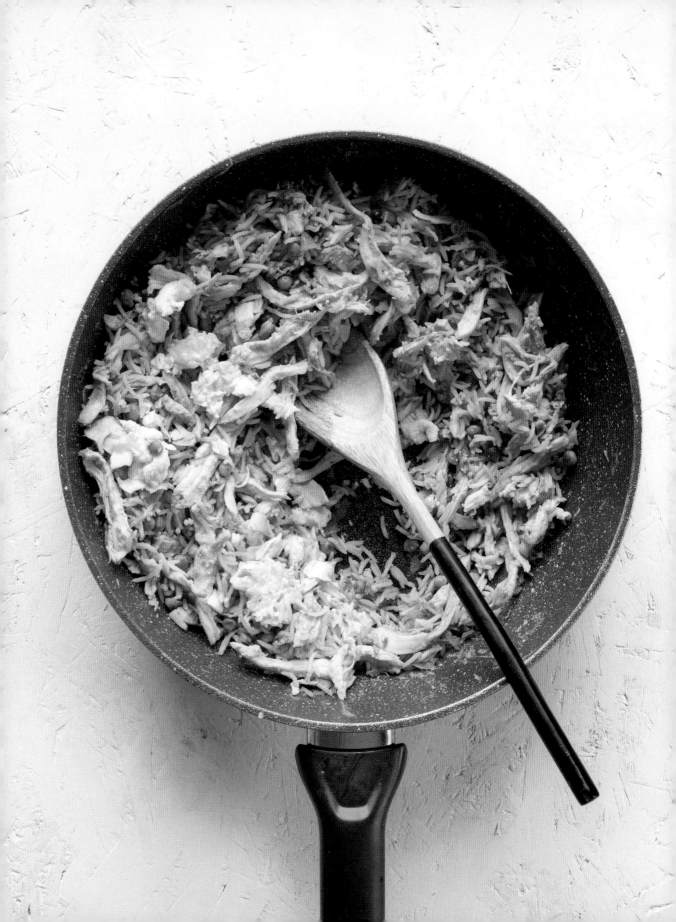

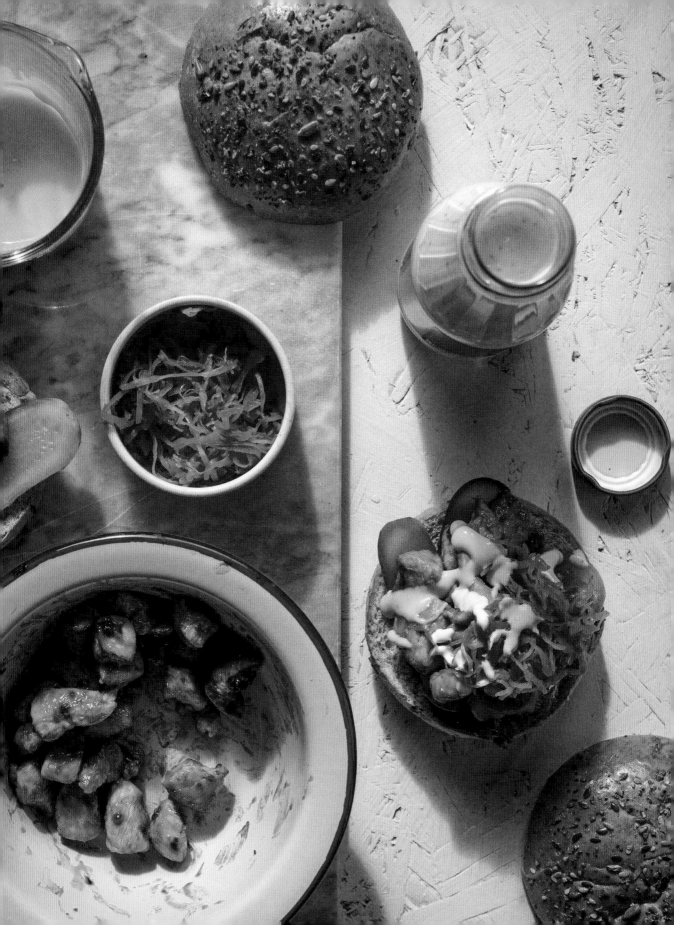

Sticky

CHICKEN BURGER

This sweet and spicy burger is very masso indeed – it's got all the flavours and taste you'd expect from a burger joint but 100 times better!

SERVES 2

Low-calorie spray oil

2 chicken breasts, chopped

2 tbsp sweet chilli sauce

2 tbsp buffalo hot sauce

3 light cheese singles, torn

2 wholemeal burger buns

1 pickled gherkin, chopped

1 jar of pickled slaw (available in supermarkets)

2 tsp shop-bought Caesar dressing

1 Spray a large wok with some oil and place over a medium heat. Add in the chopped chicken and cook, stirring regularly, until nice and brown.

2 Add in the sweet chilli sauce and toss the chicken in it until its starts to go yummy and sticky.

3 Remove from the heat, add in the buffalo sauce and give it a good mix.

4 Put the cheese singles in a small pot over a medium heat with 50ml of water and stir until blended into a smooth cheese sauce..

5 Toast the burger buns and on one half of each bun put the gherkin, then a layer of the chicken. Drizzle over the masso cheese sauce, followed by some Caesar dressing and as much pickled slaw as you like. Finish by popping the other half of the bun on top.

Crispy Tikka
CHICKEN KEBABS

Something a little different to sink your teeth into, these are great to cook in the airfryer, the oven or even on the BBQ. It's a nice all-rounder that can be kept in the fridge to throw into a salad or a wrap, a tasty little low-fat dish. You'll need four bamboo skewers to prepare this recipe, widely available in Asian markets.

SERVES 4

6 tbsp fat-free Greek yoghurt

2 garlic cloves, minced

3 tbsp tikka spice mix

4 large chicken breasts, chopped into cubes

50g instant mash (in its dry form)

½ tsp garlic granules

1 green pepper, deseeded and chopped

Salt to taste

To serve:

Wholemeal wraps

Shredded lettuce

Mango chutney

1 You'll need to start this recipe either the day before or a few hours before you want to eat it. So, mix the yoghurt, garlic, two tablespoons of the tikka spice and a grind of salt in a bowl, add in the chicken and mix well. Cover with cling film and leave in the fridge to marinate and tenderise for 2–3 hours or overnight.

2 Preheat the oven to 200°C.

3 To make the coating, mix the instant mash, the rest of the tikka spice mix, garlic granules and salt to taste in a small bowl and leave to one side.

4 Soak the skewers in water to stop them from burning when cooking, then thread cubes of chicken onto each one with a piece of green pepper between cube until you have 4 to 5 pieces of chicken on each.

5 Lay the skewers out on a baking tray. Sprinkle the instant mash mix over each skewer and shake off the excess. Pop into the preheated oven for 25–30 minutes, turning halfway through to ensure even cooking. By this time, the coating should be nice and golden and crispy.

6 Remove and place on a serving plate. Have some warmed wholemeal wraps, shredded lettuce and mango chutney at the ready for everyone to build their own crunchy tikka wraps.

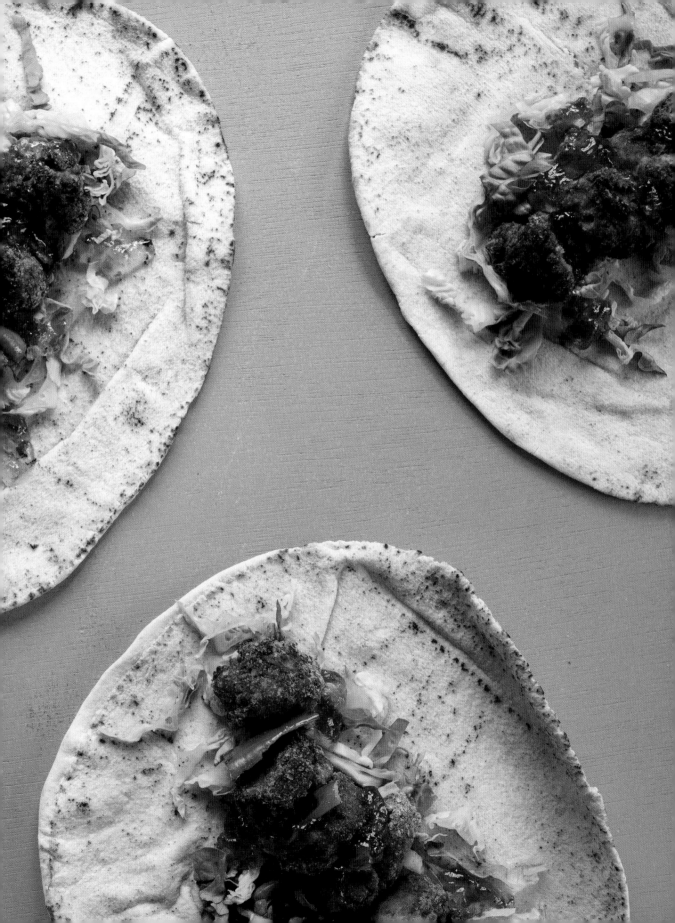

SAVAGE SNACKS

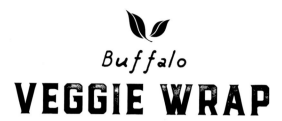

Buffalo VEGGIE WRAP

This was one of the most remade wraps from my online recipes, and you'll know why when you try it. I used shop-bought frozen vegetarian crispy nuggets for convenience but you can use regular chicken nuggets too. If you're tired of the same boring wraps and struggle to keep things interesting, this one will knock your socks off.

SERVES 1

4 vegetarian crispy nuggets

1 high-fibre wrap of your choice

15g low-fat Cheddar cheese, grated

2 tbsp tinned sweetcorn, drained

15g blue cheese, such as Cashel Blue

2 tbsp buffalo hot sauce

Iceberg lettuce, shredded

1 tbsp light Caesar sauce

1 If not using an airfryer, preheat oven to 200°C.

2 First pop the nuggets on a tray into the preheated oven or pop in the airfryer at 200°C for 10–15 minutes until golden and crisp.

3 Lay out the wrap and sprinkle over the Cheddar, sweetcorn and blue cheese.

4 Remove your nuggets from the oven or airfryer, slice in half and transfer to a small bowl. Mix with the buffalo hot sauce until evenly coated.

5 Add these to the wrap, top with some iceberg lettuce, and wrap it up.

6 Warm up a non-stick frying pan and place the wrap, folded side down, on the heat for 1–2 minutes, then flip over and repeat, which will allow the cheese to melt beautifully.

7 Remove for the heat, cut in half and serve with some Caesar sauce drizzled over.

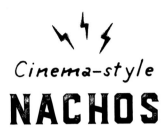

Cinema-style
NACHOS

I won't lie, I have been known to go to the cinema just for the popcorn and the nachos, wouldn't even matter what the movie was, I was just there for the treats. I'm going to show you how to make those amazing cinema-style nachos at home, with none of the guilt that goes with them.

SERVES 2

For the tortilla chips:

Low-calorie spray oil

2 wholemeal wraps

1 tbsp savoury yeast flakes

½ tsp smoked paprika

¼ tsp garlic granules

¼ tsp chilli powder

¼ tsp onion granules

Salt to taste

For the nacho sauce:

6 light cheese singles, torn

1 tsp buffalo hot sauce

To garnish:

Jalapeños (from a jar)

1 Spray some oil into a non-stick pan and place over a high heat. Pop on the first wrap, leave for 2–3 minutes, then flip and fry the other side. Remove from the pan and leave to cool on a wire rack. Repeat with the second wrap.

2 Put the rest of the tortilla ingredients in a pestle and mortar and bash until crushed.

3 For the nacho sauce, put the light cheese singles in a small pot with 50ml of water over a medium heat. Stir until smooth, then add the buffalo hot sauce and mix well.

4 Take the cooked wraps and place on a board. Spray a little oil in the middle of each and then rub in all over with your hand. Sprinkle over your seasoning (it will stick to the oil) and shake off the excess.

5 Finish by using a pizza cutter to cut the wraps into triangles and shake off the excess seasoning.

6 Pour the cheese sauce into a ramekin and get dipping and crunching! Serve with some jalapeños on the side.

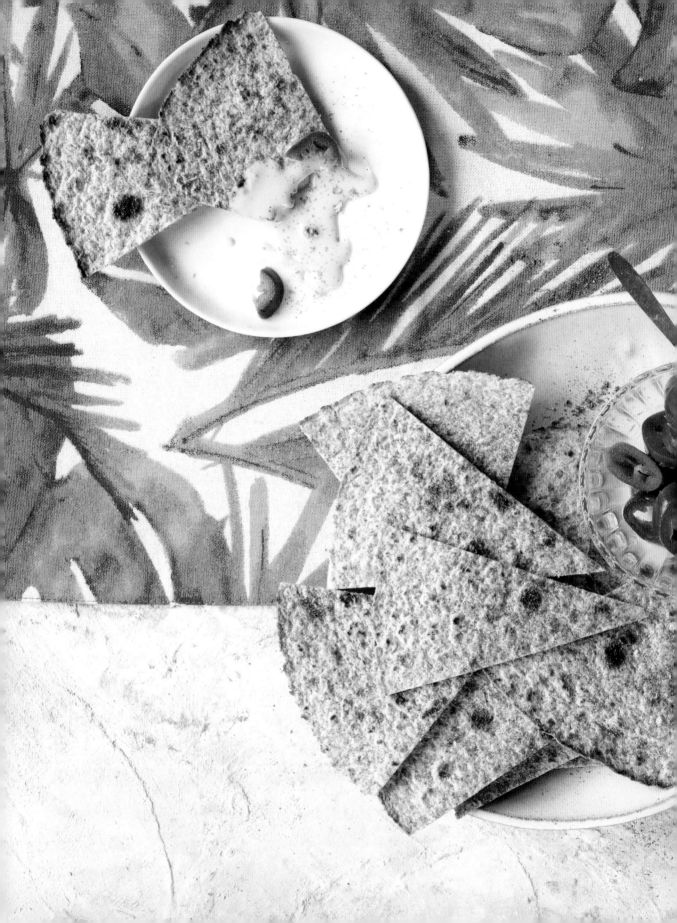

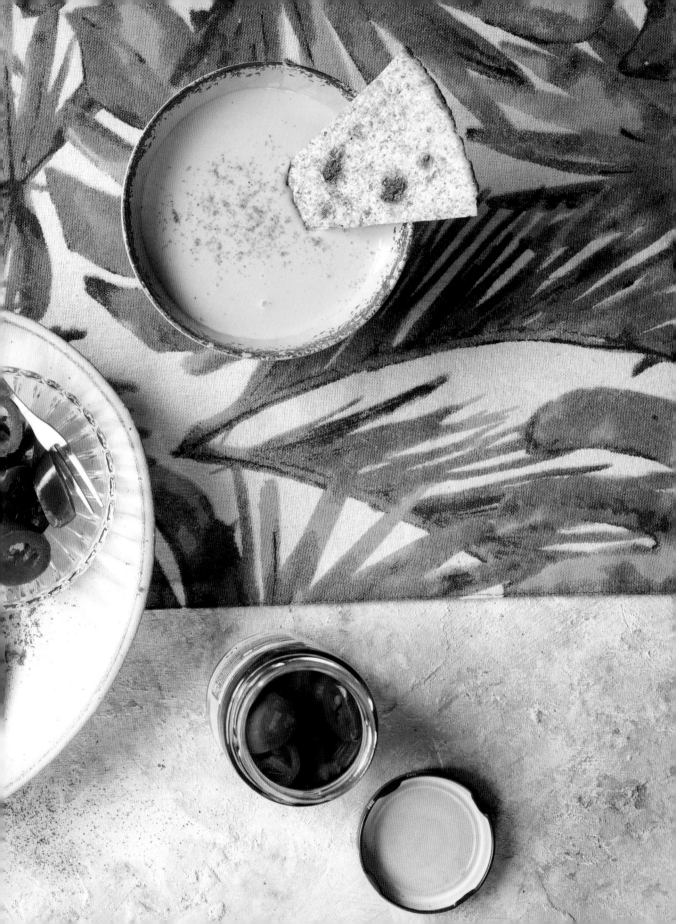

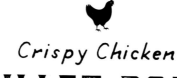

Crispy Chicken

FILLET ROLL

No more trips to the deli needed – I've got you covered with this tasty lunch treat. Crispy chicken in a roll or bread of your choice drizzled with satay sauce and loaded with fresh crisp iceberg lettuce, the ultimate day after the night before dream snack.

SERVES 1

10g panko breadcrumbs

1 tsp lemon pepper

1 egg, beaten

1 chicken fillet

1 high-fibre wholemeal roll

1 tbsp lighter mayonnaise

¼ tsp white pepper

Iceberg lettuce, torn

1 tomato, sliced

1 If not using an airfryer, preheat your oven to 200°C.

2 Mix the panko breadcrumbs with the lemon pepper in one bowl and pour the beaten egg into another bowl. Dunk the chicken fillet into the egg, shake off excess, then dip into the panko mix until evenly coated.

3 Pop into the airfryer at 180°C for 15–20 minutes until golden and crispy, turning halfway through. You can also cook on a tray in a preheated oven for 25 minutes. Remove and slice (or leave whole if you prefer)

4 Slice the roll in half and toast lightly in the oven or under a grill. Mix the mayo with the white pepper and spoon it onto the bottom part of the roll.

5 Add the lettuce and slices of tomato, then the sliced crispy chicken and wrap your chops around that deli-style treat created in your very own kitchen.

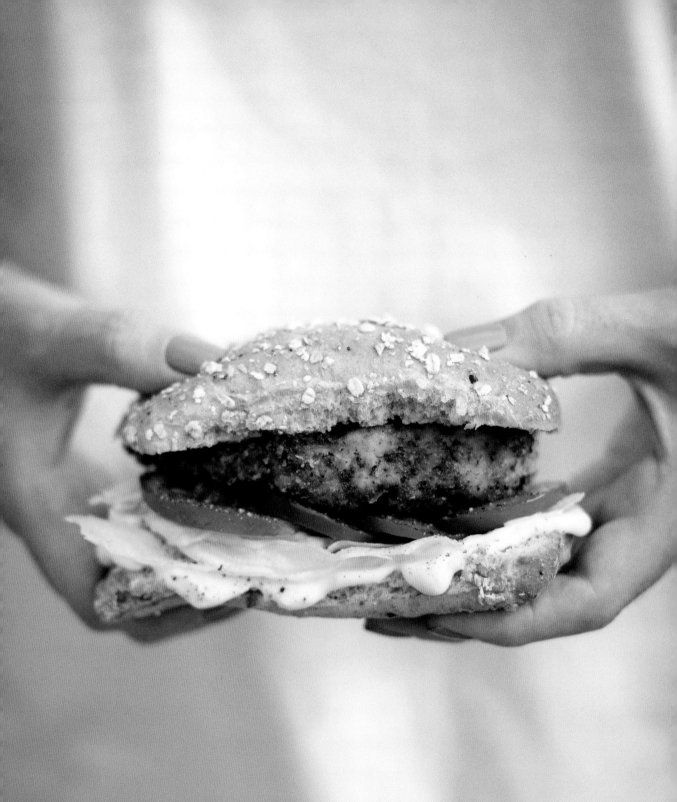

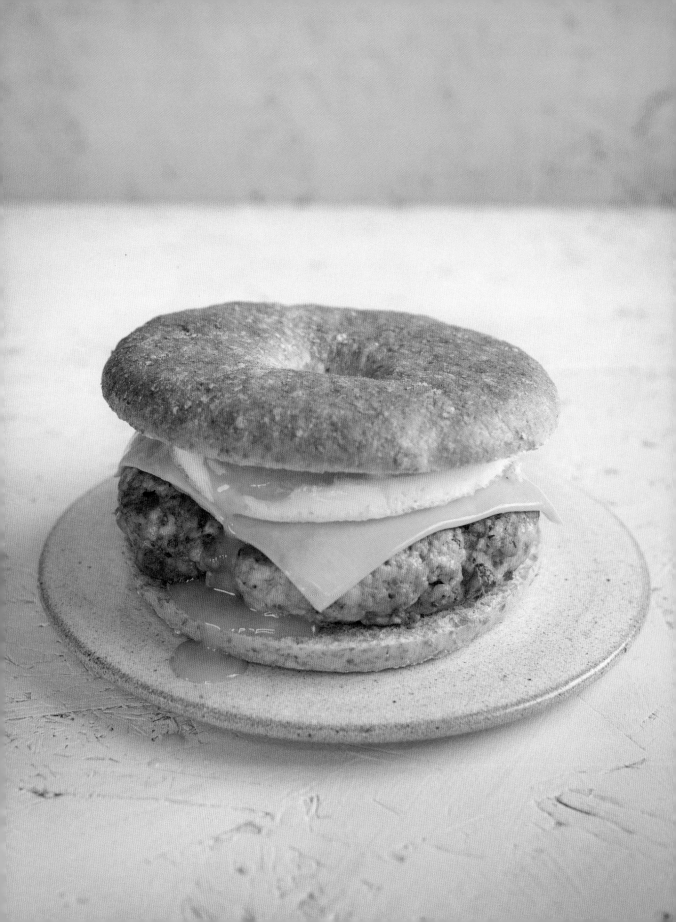

Sausage and Egg Muffin
FROM SCRATCH

From the comfort of your own gaff! Hun bun and pyjamas are essential in the making of this breakfast feast.

SERVES 4

For the patties:

400 g lean pork mince

1 tsp dried sage

½ tsp mixed herbs

½ tsp white pepper

Salt to taste

For the other bits:

4 eggs

4 wholemeal muffins/bagel thins, halved

4 light cheese singles

1 Put the mince in a bowl with the with the spices and a pinch of salt, get your (clean) hands in there and give it a good aul mix.

2 Shape into four patties roughly the size of your palm. I like mine thin so I flatten them really well.

3 Heat a non-stick pan on a medium heat and add the patties, cook for 5–6 minutes per side (depending on the thickness) until golden brown, then remove from pan and leave to one side.

4 In the same pan, crack in your eggs. If you want them perfectly round use an egg mould to keep the edges in, but I'm not fussed.

5 Pop a drop of water in the pan, cover with a lid and leave for 3 minutes – this will fry and poach them at the same time and cook the top.

6 Toast the muffins/bagel thins, to one half add a sausage patty, a slice of cheese, then an egg, top with the other half and boom, you have yourself an epic breakfast.

7 Serve with one of my Dishy Hash Browns (page 102) for the full experience.

Dishy
HASH BROWNS

Who doesn't love a deadly hash brown? These little beauties are so easy to make, with none of the hassle of grating! You'll wonder how you ever lived without them. These are both airfryer– and oven–friendly.

SERVES 2

2–3 large potatoes, peeled and chopped into quarters

Low-calorie spray oil

1 medium onion, finely chopped

Salt and pepper to taste

½ tsp smoked/regular paprika

1 If not using an airfryer, preheat your oven to 200°C. Place your potatoes in a microwave-safe bowl and cook in the microwave for about 8–10 minutes, until soft – they should be almost mashable but not mushy and still firm enough to chop up.

2 Heat a non-stick pan with a spray of oil and fry off the chopped onion until translucent.

3 Once the potatoes are microwaved, allow to cool for 5–10 minutes then chop into small cubes or mash roughly with a fork. Put the cubes in a bowl, tip in the cooked onion, then add some salt, pepper and the smoked/regular paprika.

4 With clean hands, take a palm-sized piece of the mixture, pat together into a hash brown shape and place on a plate nearby. Continue until you've used up all the mixture. Once they are ready, spray lightly with oil and pop in your airfryer for 15 minutes at 190°C, turning a couple of times and respraying. They should look golden brown when finished.

5 If oven cooking, place on a baking tray, spray with oil and cook in the preheated oven for 15–30 minutes, checking along the way and turning.

6 Plate up and sprinkle a little extra paprika for a pop of taste and colour.

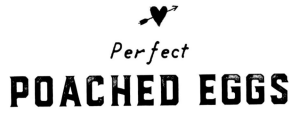

Perfect
POACHED EGGS

Poached eggs on toast, an absolute classic! If you struggle to get the perfect poached egg here is how I make mine and they never disappoint. The trick is to add some vinegar to the water, which firms up the white quicker and stops it getting lost in the water. Also, don't overfill the pot or the egg will travel around like a mad thing!

SERVES 1

1 egg
2 tsp white/malt vinegar

To serve:

Toast and butter

1 Crack the egg into a small ramekin.

2 Pour 3–4 inches of boiling water from the kettle into a small saucepan and pop it on a medium heat – you don't want the water to be bubbling because this will push the eggs around and you'll lose some of the white.

3 Add in the vinegar, and with the end of a wooden spoon stir the water in one direction until you have a little vortex going on in the centre.

4 Gently drop the egg in – the spinning will allow the white to form around the yolk.

5 Cook for 3 minutes until the white has firmed up, then remove from the heat.

6 Butter up some toast and put the egg on top. I like to pierce mine with a sharp knife and let the yolk ooze out deliciously over the buttery toast.

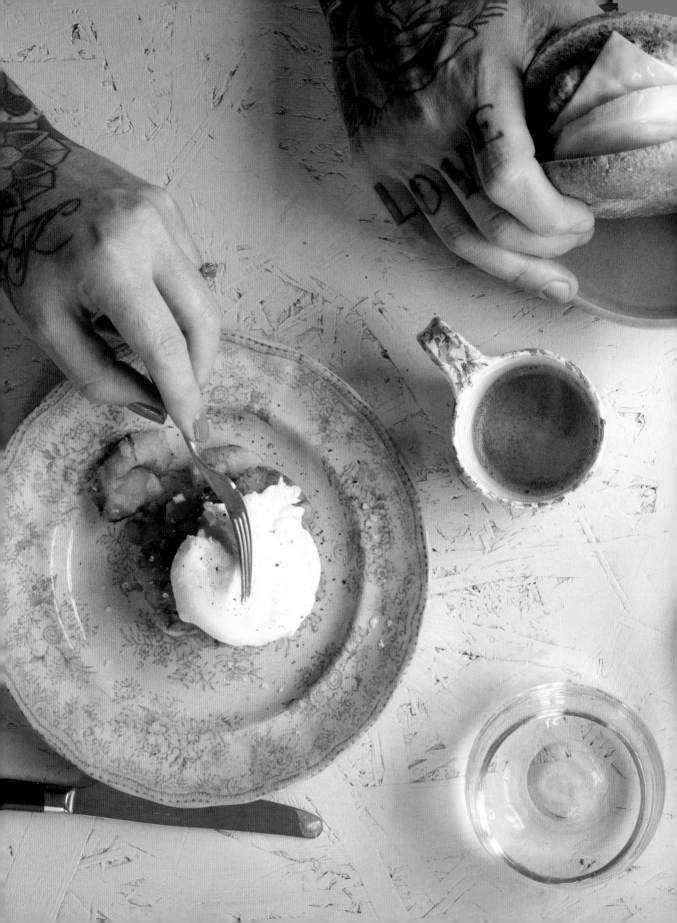

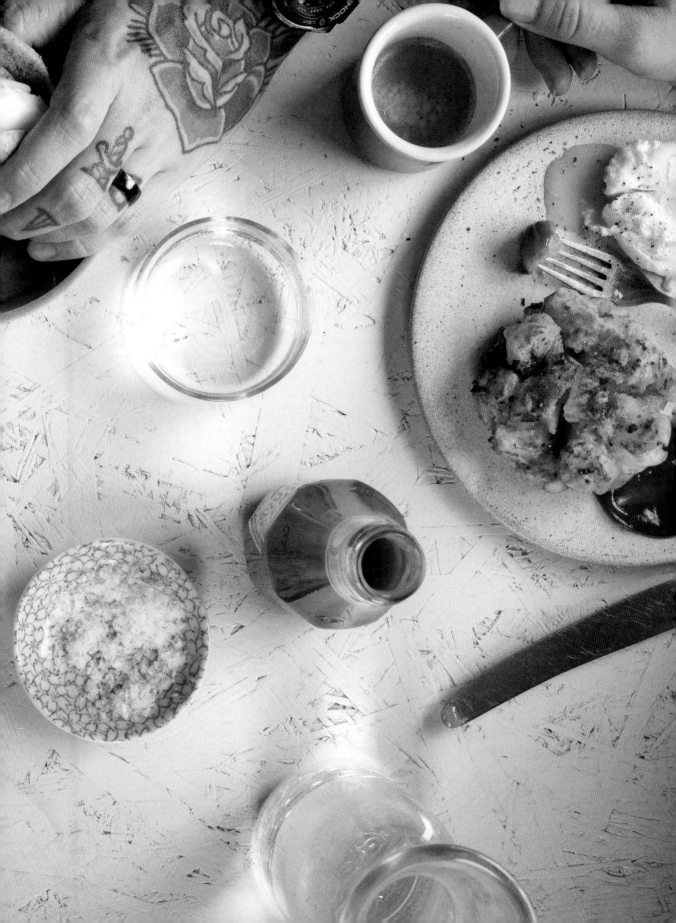

On-the-pan

CHEESE TOASTIE

A cheese toastie is one of the best comfort foods ever. I never owned a sandwich maker and always struggled to get toasties just right under the grill so I started popping them on the frying pan and the rest is history! You can fill them with whatever filling you like but this is my favourite combination.

SERVES 1

2 slices (60g) sliced wholemeal bread

40g low-fat Cheddar cheese, grated

½ a medium tomato, sliced

Ham or prosciutto (optional)

Low-calorie spray oil

1 On a board, lay out one of the slices of bread and add 25g of the Cheddar, the sliced tomato and the ham (if you fancy a bit of meat). Pop the second slice on top and squish slightly.

2 Heat a non-stick frying pan on a medium heat, spray with 5 sprays of oil, place the sambo in the pan and allow to cook for 4–5 minutes to crisp up the bottom part.

3 Spray the top of the bread with another 5 sprays of oil, flip over and cook for another 4–5 minutes.

4 When both sides are cooked, remove the toastie and sprinkle the remaining cheese on the hot pan. When it starts to sizzle, sit the toastie on top of the cheese and leave for up to 1 minute.

5 Lift out of the pan cheese side facing up – you should have a nice melted inside and a lovely cheese crust on the outside.

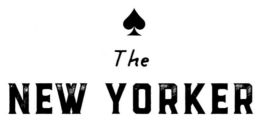

The

NEW YORKER

I visited New York for a few days back in 2006 when my friend was on a working visa. New York blew my mind. Yes, the buildings and sights were incredible but my Jaysus the food blew my mind even more. Before my flight home I picked up a sambo from a deli and it was incredible. I used to think about it all the time, so inevitably I had to recreate it.

SERVES 2

500g potatoes, peeled and cut into chips

Low-calorie spray oil

2 wholemeal bagel slims, halved

2 pickled gherkins, sliced thinly

130g peppered pastrami

30g low-fat Cheddar cheese, grated

2 tbsp American yellow mustard

1 If not using an airfryer, preheat your oven to 220°C.

2 First sort your fries out: follow the instructions for Perfect Chips on page 44.

3 Toast the bagels and add a layer of the sliced pickled gherkin to the bottom half of each one. Next pile up your pastrami, the more the better. Grab a handful of the fries and load them on there too.

4 Sprinkle the cheese on top and pop into the airfyer or under the grill until the cheese melts.

5 Drizzle some mustard over the top and pop on the top half of the bagel.

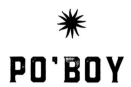

PO'BOY

A po'boy is a traditional roll-like sandwich from Louisiana. The filling of deep-fried shrimps and salad is served on a baguette and topped with remoulade sauce. Here is my version of a po'boy without the need for deep frying and with a homemade sauce to drizzle over the top.

SERVES 2

40g instant mash (in its dry form)

½ tsp smoked paprika

½ tsp garlic granules

1 tsp lemon pepper

200g prawns, raw and peeled

1 egg, beaten

Low-calorie spray oil

For the sauce:

3 tbsp lighter than light mayo

1 tsp yellow American mustard

1 pickled gherkin, finely chopped

1 tsp pickle juice from gherkin jar

1 garlic clove, finely minced

Juice of ½ a lime

For the roll:

2 wholemeal hot dog rolls

1 tomato, sliced

Shredded lettuce

1 Preheat the oven to 180°C.

2 Pop the instant mash and the three spices into a bowl and mix well.

3 Put the beaten egg in a separate bowl, then dip the prawns one by one into the egg, then into the spice mix, making sure all the prawns are coated evenly.

4 Spray a baking tray with a little oil and lay the coated prawns out on it.

5 Cook in the preheated oven for 15 minutes, turning and spraying with a little oil halfway through until the coating is golden brown.

6 Mix the six ingredients for the sauce in a small bowl and put to one side.

7 Slice the rolls in half and pop into the oven for the last three minutes until heated through.

8 Now it's time to assemble your po'boys: layer the rolls with the tomato and lettuce, divide the crispy prawns between them and drizzle over the sauce.

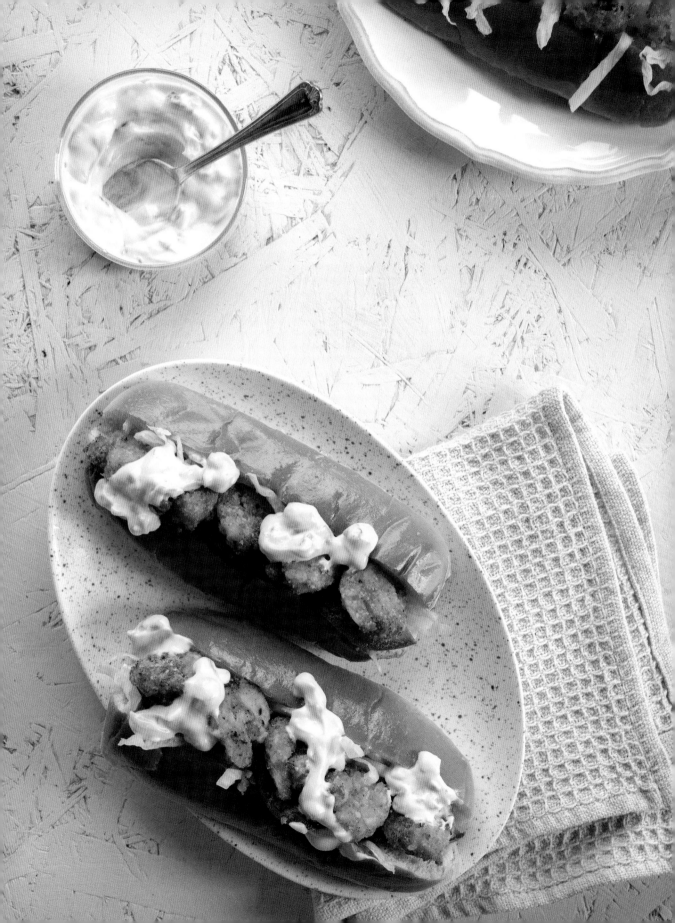

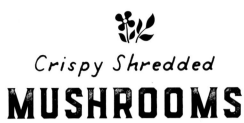

Crispy Shredded
MUSHROOMS

These work so well as an alternative to meat and are super tasty and so handy to make. I serve mine with a deadly little sticky garlic and soy sauce. Delish!

SERVES 4

8 large portobello mushrooms
Low-calorie spray oil
6 tbsp cornflour
150ml rapeseed oil

For the sticky soy and ginger sauce:

100ml soy sauce
2 tbsp sweet chilli sauce
1 garlic clove, crushed
½ tsp ground ginger
½ tsp sesame seeds

To serve:

Basmati rice
1 fresh red chilli, chopped
1 spring onion, chopped

1 If not using an airfryer, preheat your oven to 180°C.

2 Clean off the mushrooms and pop them whole into your airfryer with a spray of oil at 180°C for 10 minutes, or in the preheated oven for 15 minutes. Once they are ready, slice them up into strips.

3 Put the cornflour in a medium-sized bowl and add in the mushrooms. Toss them around until they are fully coated in the cornflour.

4 Grab a wok or non-stick pan and pour in the rapeseed oil. Don't worry too much about using the oil as most of it will stay behind in the pan after cooking and we will be patting the excess off. Bring up the heat to allow the oil to get nice and hot, then add in the coated mushrooms. They should start to sizzle and the flour will begin to go nice and crispy. They will only need a few minutes in the pan to get the desired crispiness and this is the point where you will get very excited because they will look only gorgeous! When they are ready remove from the wok or pan, place on some kitchen paper and pat off any excess oil.

5 To make the sticky sauce, put the soy in a saucepan with the chilli sauce, crushed garlic and ground ginger. Bring up the heat and stir everything together until thickened (about 2–3 minutes). The aromas will be unreal! Now throw in the crispy mushrooms and toss around in the sauce until they are completely covered. Plate them babies up and sprinkle with some sesame seeds. I like to serve mine on a bed of rice and garnish with fresh chillies and spring onion. You'll wonder where they have been all your life.

♥

The

DALY DOG

I absolutely love hot dogs but if I'm honest I rarely eat them! I have this thing in my head that I just can't shake, about not knowing what's inside them – slightly dramatic I know, but that's why I created these. Now I know for sure what's in every bite. You'll need to start this recipe a couple of hours before you want to eat it.

Serves 4-6

500g lean beef mince

100g chorizo, chopped

1 tsp dark soy sauce

½ tsp chilli flakes (if you want it spicy)

½ tsp garlic powder

10 green jalapeños, finely chopped (from a jar)

1 tbsp tomato purée

1 tsp smoked paprika

1 tbsp buffalo hot sauce

½ tsp mixed herbs

Low-calorie spray oil

For the topping:

6 light cheese singles, torn

4-6 wholemeal hot dog buns

1 onion, finely chopped

1 Get a large bowl and throw in all the 'sausage' ingredients (except the oil). Give it a good aul stir then cover and leave in the fridge for 1–2 hours to let all the flavours mix well.

2 With clean hands, take palm-sized pieces of the mince mixture, squeeze out the excess liquid, form in to a ball then lay on a piece of greaseproof paper. Start to roll each ball out into a sausage shape and size.

3 Repeat until you use up all the mixture – you can make them as big or as small as you like.

4 Spray some oil into a non-stick pan and cook your sausages until they are nice and golden brown; they will be delicate so handle them with care.

5 To make the cheese sauce, melt the cheese slices in a small pot with 100ml water until smooth.

6 Toast your buns and pop in your sausage, pour over the cheese sauce and garnish with the onion.

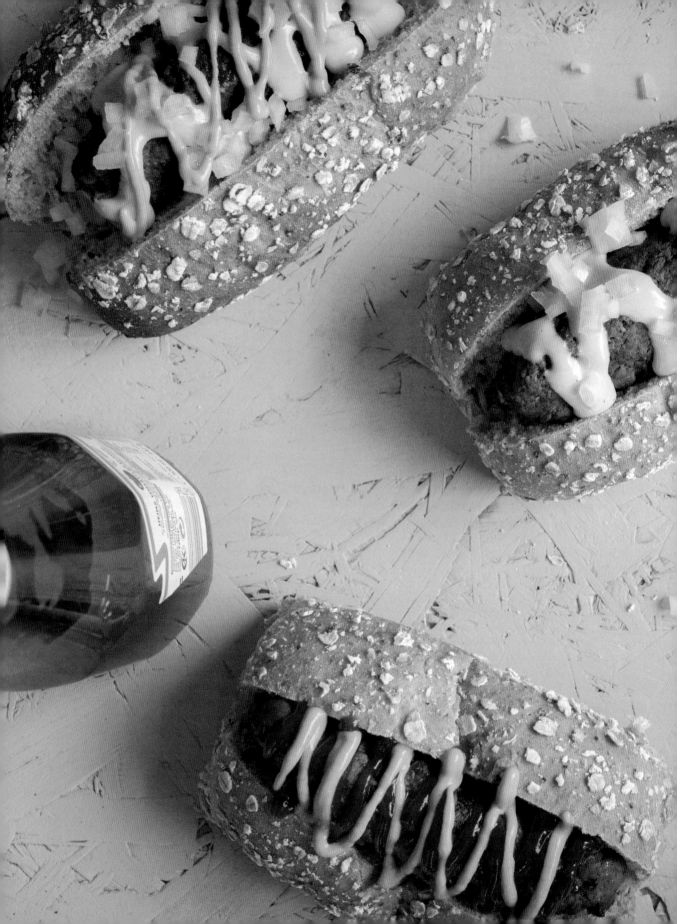

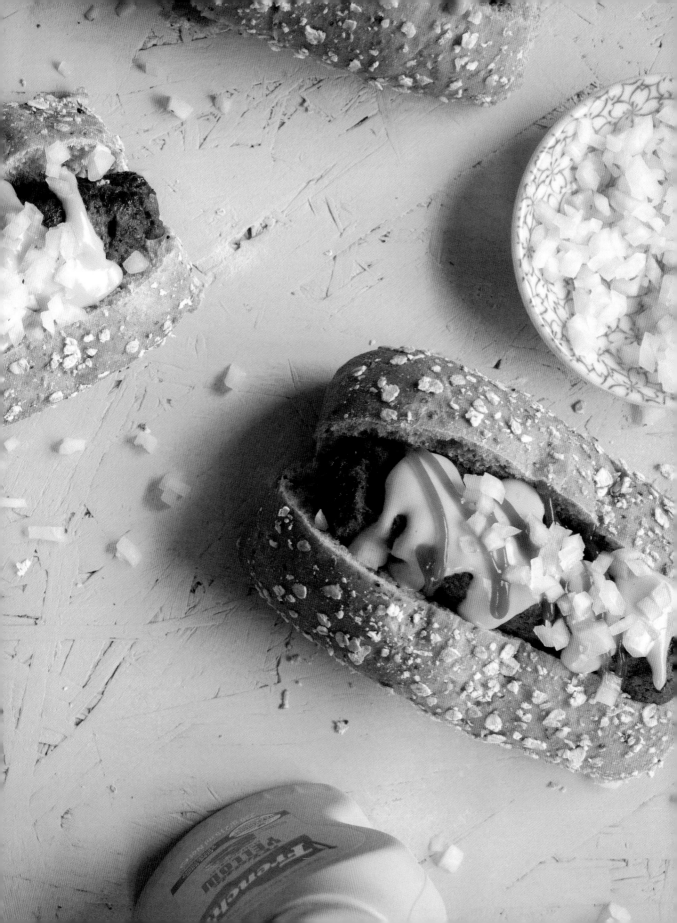

Cheese and Onion
CRISPS

My biggest guilty pleasure is a nice bag of cheese and onion crisps, especially when they are slapped between two slices of bread. I tried for ages to get the right flavour and then boom, I had an epiphany and these little beauties were born. None of the grease and all of the flavour. Batch cook them and keep them in an airtight container to have as an evening snack or on the side, deli-style, with a nice healthy wrap.

SERVES 4

500g new potatoes, washed and peeled

Low-calorie spray oil

1 tbsp savoury yeast flakes

1 tbsp onion granules

1 If not using an airfryer, preheat your oven to 220°C. Using a sharp knife, slice your spuds into thin, crisp-like slices, rinse then drain all the water, put in a microwave-safe bowl and pop in the microwave for 6–7 minutes until slightly soft.

2 Remove, spray lightly with oil and pop on a tray and into a preheated oven at 220°C for 15–20 minutes. If using an airfryer pop them in at 200°C for 15 minutes, shaking and respraying halfway through.

3 Put the yeast flakes and onion granules in a pestle and mortar and give them a good grind until reduced to a fine powder. You will only use a small amount of this seasoning so you can save the rest in an airtight container for the next batch.

4 When your crisps are ready transfer into a bowl with about 4 teaspoons of the seasoning and toss to combine. For that packet-of-crisps vibe you could portion them out into four paper bags and add half a teaspoon of the seasoning to each portion, giving them a good shake to coat the crisps well. Either way, enjoy every bite!

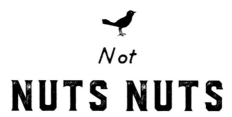

Not

NUTS NUTS

If you love a little snack of something to nibble on while watching a movie these will be right up your street. You can be as adventurous as you like with the spices and seasoning but this little recipe will get you started.

SERVES 2-3

1 x 400g tin of chickpeas, drained

1 tsp smoked paprika

1 tsp garlic granules

1 tsp onion granules

Low-calorie spray oil

Salt to taste

1 If not using an airfryer, preheat the oven to 200°C.

2 Pop the chickpeas into a bowl, shake over the paprika, garlic granules and onion granules and stir well to make sure the chickpeas are evenly coated.

3 Lay the coated chickpeas on a baking sheet, spray 5-6 times with the spray oil and put in the preheated oven for 35–40 minutes, turning and respraying halfway through until golden and crisp.

4 If using an airfryer, pop them in at 190°C for 15–20 minutes with a spray of oil, shaking and respraying halfway through.

5 Remove the crispy little balls of loveliness and sprinkle with a little salt to taste.

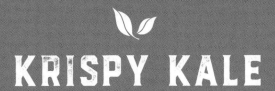

KRISPY KALE

Kale is one of the world's 'superfoods' – it's full of antioxidants, nutrients and all that jazz. However, it's not one that ever really appealed to me. Over the years I've really tried to add more fruit and vegetables to my diet so I wanted to make it appeal and be something I wanted to eat. Below is the answer!

SERVES 4

250g fresh kale
1 tsp lemon pepper
15g Parmesan cheese, grated
Low-calorie spray oil

1 Preheat your oven to 150–160°C.
2 Wash the kale (I remove the stalks, because I can't be dealing with them) and dry.
3 Lay out on a large baking sheet in a single layer (you might need to use 2 trays), spray with the oil and massage it in to coat evenly.
4 Sprinkle over the lemon pepper and Parmesan cheese.
5 Pop in the oven for 15–20 minutes until nice and crisp.
6 Serve in a bowl as a tasty evening snack, or on the side with a wrap or sandwich for extra nutrition.

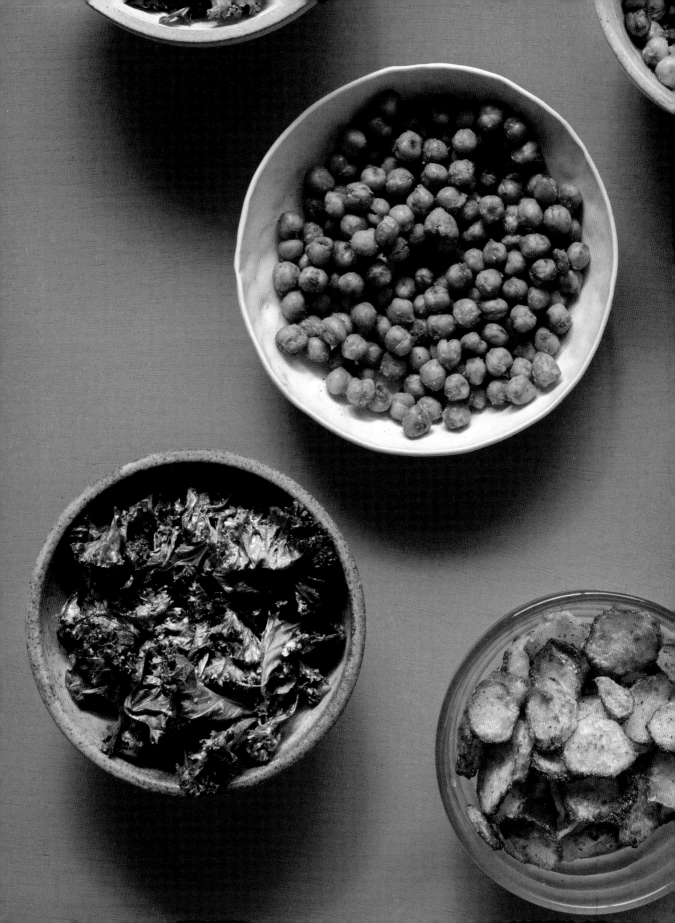

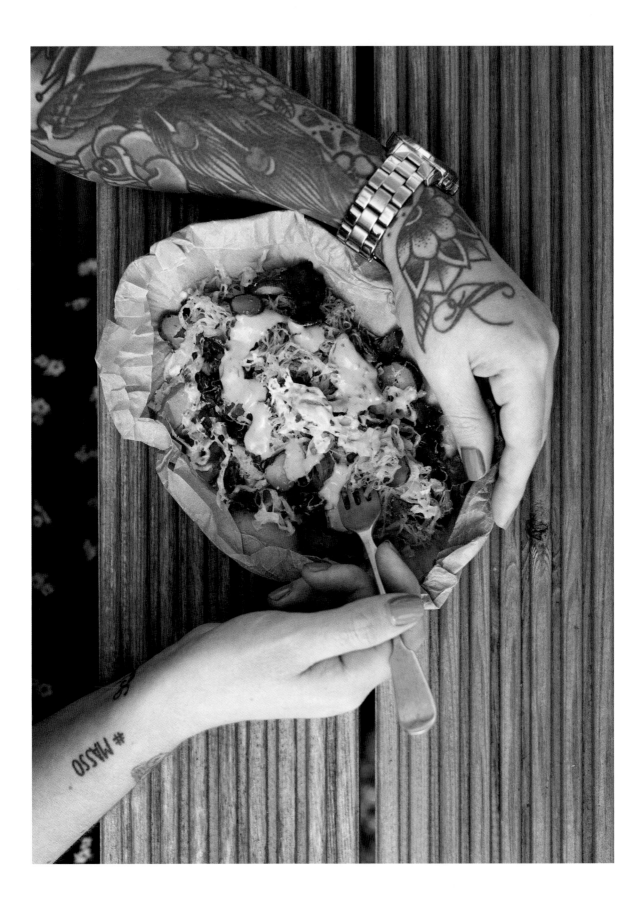

Rockin'

REUBEN SALAD

I'm not the biggest fan of lettuce in a salad. I really wish I loved it as it would've made my lunch options so much easier over the years and probably stopped me reaching for the less healthy choices. Anyway, I found an alternative that I liked and made this fab salad that is now a regular on my lunch menu.

SERVES 1

3 generous tbsp of pickled sauerkraut (from a jar)

½ tsp lemon pepper

50g pastrami, torn

1 pickled gherkin, sliced

30g low-fat Cheddar cheese, grated

1 tbsp light thousand island dressing

1 Put the sauerkraut and lemon pepper in a warm pan and fry off for 2–3 minutes.

2 Throw in the pastrami and pickled gherkin and let it all fry for another 2–3 minutes.

3 Transfer the mix to the middle of a sheet of greaseproof paper and roll in the sides until it's like a little bowl, then sprinkle the cheese over the top.

4 Pop it under a hot grill or alternatively pop it in to the airfryer at 180°C for 4–5 minutes until the cheese melts.

5 For a fuss-free lunch drizzle the thousand island dressing straight over the top and dive straight in eating right out of the paper – saves on the washing up too! Win-win.

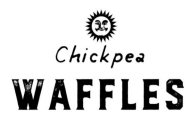

Chickpea WAFFLES

Chickpeas are great things altogether. You can use them for practically anything at all – everything from hummus to a curry. These little bites of joy are another great way to get the most out of chickpeas. You'll need a waffle maker to make this recipe.

SERVES 2-3

1 x 400g tin of chickpeas, drained

30g Cheddar & mozzarella cheese mix (available in super-markets)

1 egg

1 tbsp sweet chilli sauce

½ tsp smoked paprika

A pinch of salt to taste

Low-calorie spray oil

1 Put the chickpeas into a mixing bowl. Blend until smooth with a hand blender.

2 Throw in the cheese and crack in the egg along with the sweet chilli sauce and paprika and mix well with a fork until it's a dough-like consistency. Add a pinch of salt to taste.

3 With clean hands, take palm-sized pieces of the mixture and flatten into patties.

4 Heat your waffle iron, spray with the oil and pop a patty in. Close over and allow to cook for 5–6 minutes until golden brown, then repeat until you've used up all the mixture.

5 Serve with your favourite dipping sauce.

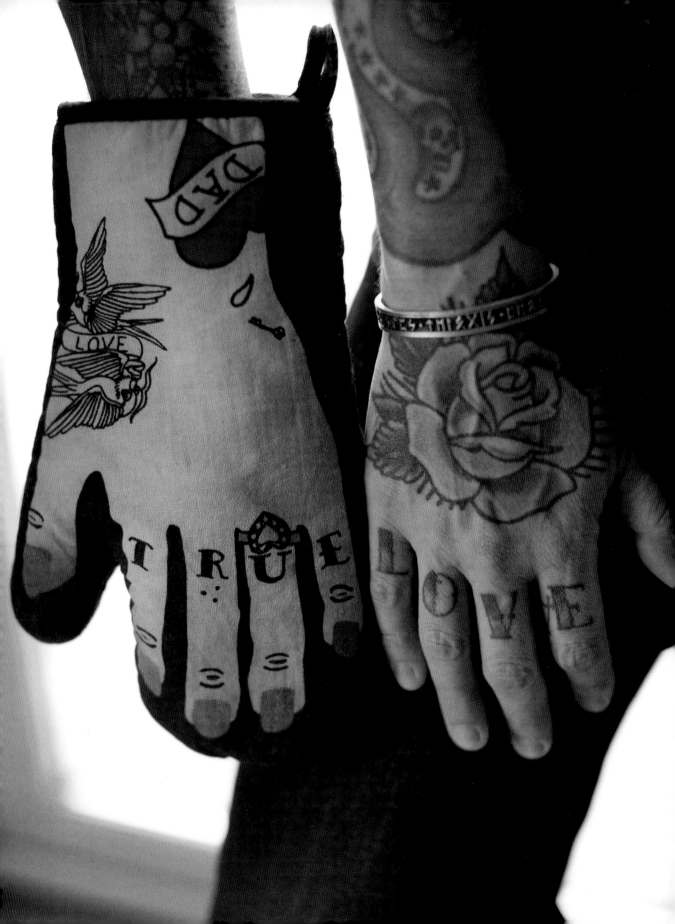

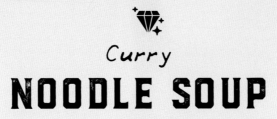

Curry
NOODLE SOUP

This warm, tasty, satisfying little gem can be ready in less than ten minutes. Handy on the days when time is of the essence and also great to batch cook and pop in a flask to take to work or school as a nutritious hot lunch.

SERVES 4

Low-calorie spray oil

1 tsp handy garlic

1 tsp handy chilli

350g frozen vegetable mix

1 tsp dark soy sauce

1 x 400g tin of no-added-sugar chicken soup

2 balls of frozen spinach

2 tsp medium curry powder

1 nest of vermicelli rice noodles

Sea salt and black pepper to taste

1 Spray your wok with some oil, add the garlic and chilli and fry off for 2–3 minutes.

2 Add in the frozen vegetables and the soy sauce and cook until the vegetables are tender.

3 Add in the tin of soup and the frozen spinach, give it all a good mix, bring up the heat then add the curry powder.

4 Blanch the vermicelli noodles in boiling water for 2 minutes until they soften, then drain and add them into the wok.

5 Give everything a good stir until the spinach is cooked. if it looks too thick at this stage you can add in some water to make the mixture more 'soupy'.

6 Once ready, serve in warm bowls, grind over some sea salt and black pepper and tuck in.

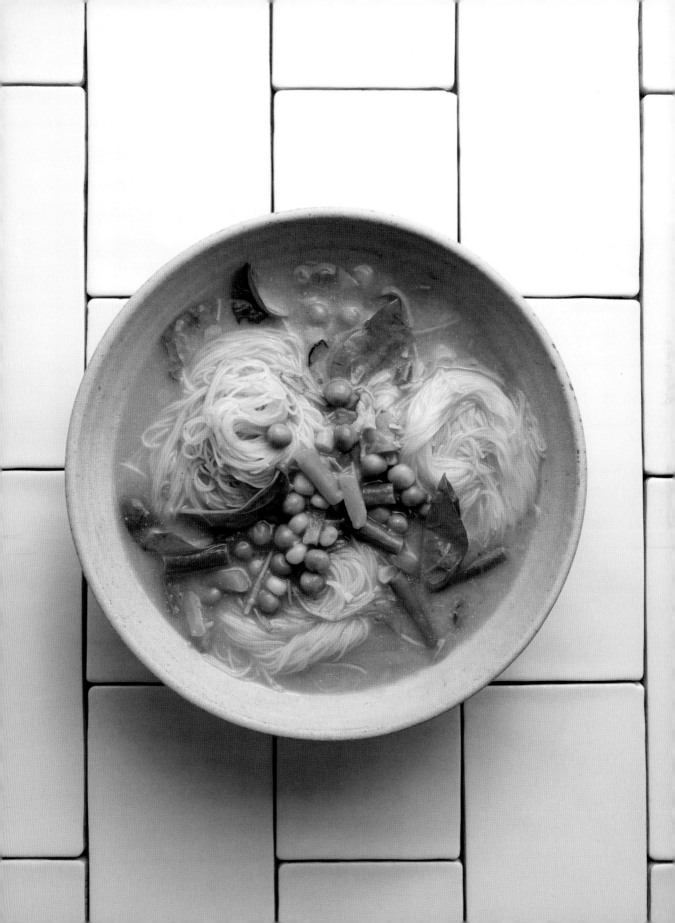

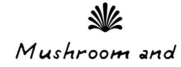

Mushroom and
ASPARAGUS SOUP

Spring, summer, autumn, winter, I LOVE soup. So handy to make, fills you up, and you can have so many combinations of flavours. This is one of my favourites, and the cheeky little bit of Parmesan is the icing on the cake.

SERVES 4

Low-calorie spray oil

3 cloves of garlic, crushed

500g mushrooms, chopped

1 onion, finely chopped

800ml chicken/vegetable stock

10 asparagus spears

60g Parmesan cheese, grated

1 Get the biggest pot you have, spray the bottom with the oil and get it nice and hot.

2 Add in the garlic and cook off for 1–2 minutes, then add in the mushrooms and onion and fry off until the onion is translucent. The mushrooms will release lots of liquid, and that's good – you want all that flavour in the soup.

3 Pour in the stock and bring it to a boil, then turn down the heat and let it simmer, covered, for 10–15 minutes.

4 Meanwhile prep the asparagus: you can boil or griddle it, or lash it in an airfryer at 180°C for 10 minutes with a spray of oil.

5 When the soup is ready remove from the heat and blend in the pot with a hand blender until smooth. Pop in the Parmesan and give it a good stir until it melts in, then chop up the cooked asparagus and pop that in too.

6 Ladle into warm bowls and finish off with an extra little sprinkle of Parmesan! Masso.

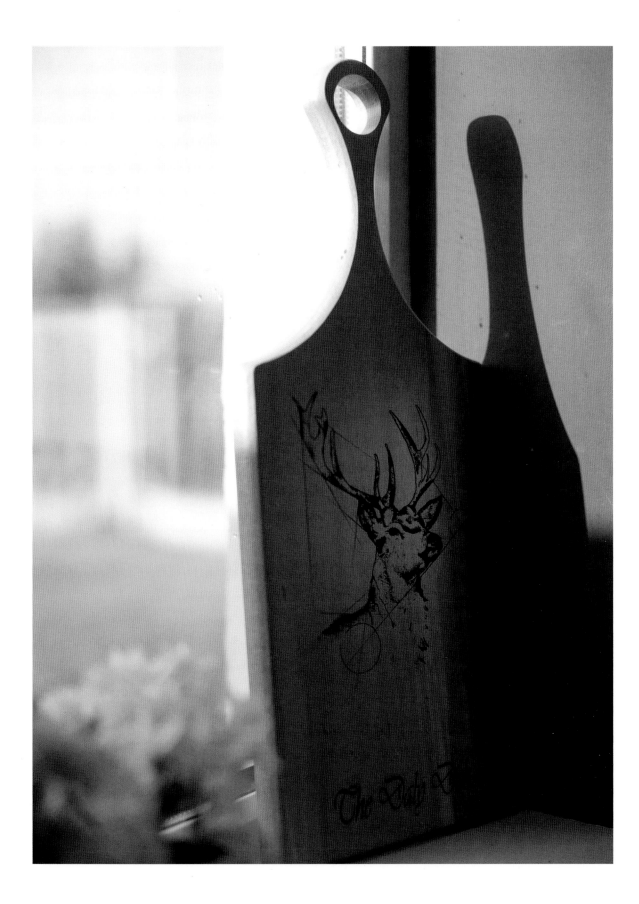

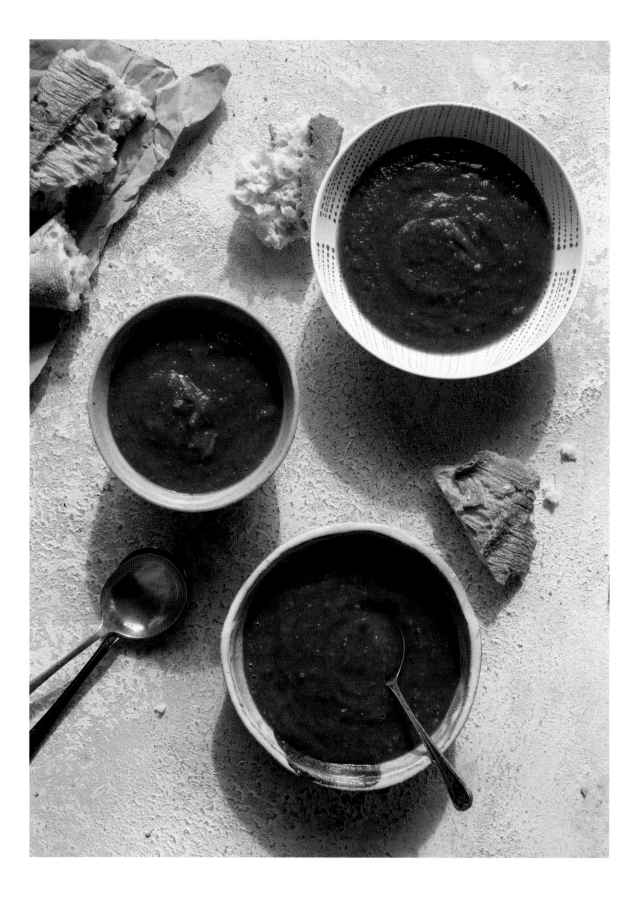

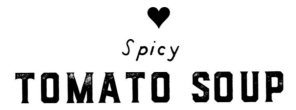

Spicy
TOMATO SOUP

This is a deadly winter warmer – lash on the PJs, stick on the heating and get this into ya!

SERVES 4

6 large tomatoes, halved

2 medium onions, halved

6 garlic cloves, peeled

Low-calorie spray oil

1 x 400g tin of chopped tomatoes

300ml vegetable stock

1 tbsp sweetener or brown sugar

1 tsp paprika

½ tsp mixed herbs

½ tsp chilli flakes (leave out if you can't handle the heat)

A dash of Worcestershire sauce

1 Preheat oven to 220°C.

2 Lay out the tomatoes, onion and garlic on a baking tray, spray lightly with oil and roast for 15–20 minutes until they start to take on some colour.

3 Place the roasted vegetables into a large pot on a medium then add in the tin of tomatoes and the vegetable stock.

4 Stir well and bring up to a boil, then reduce the heat and allow to simmer for 10 minutes.

5 Add in the rest of the ingredients and continue to simmer for another 5 minutes, then remove from the heat.

6 Pour into a blender and blitz until smooth or use a hand blender placed directly into the pot.

7 Serve in a warm bowls with a slice of crusty bread if you're feeling cheeky.

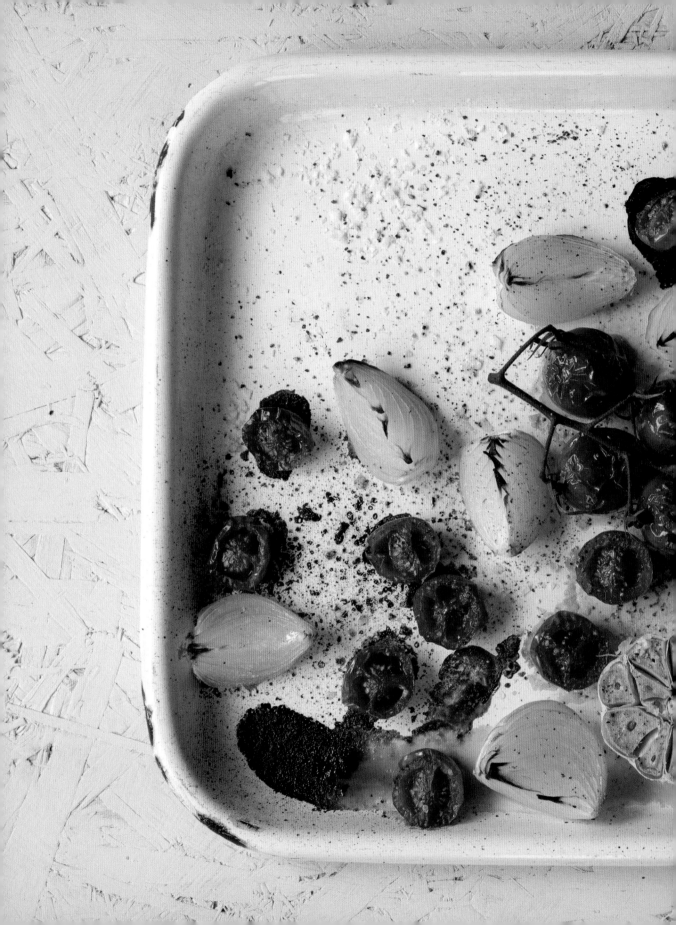

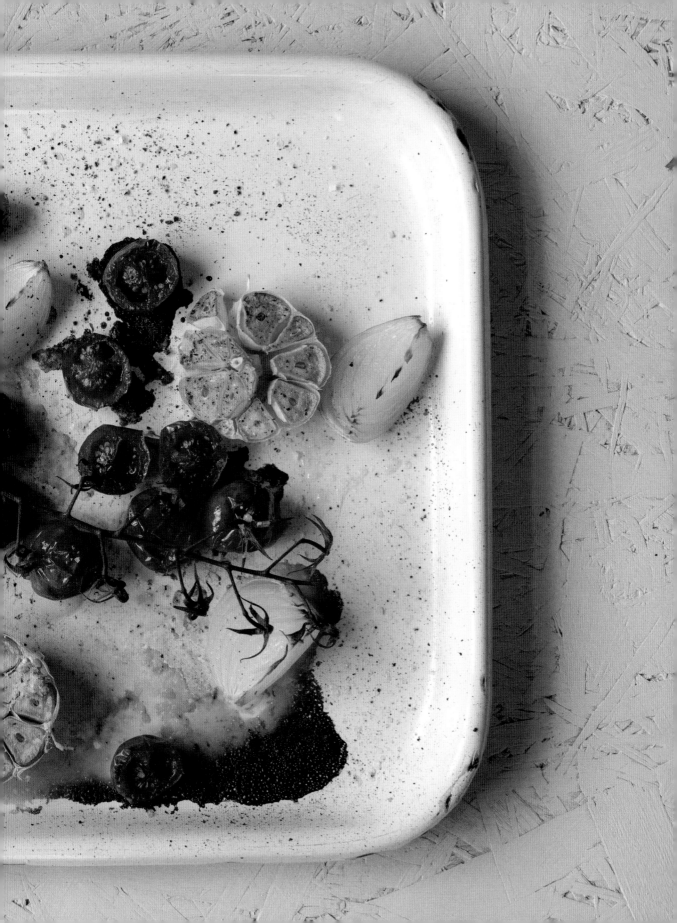

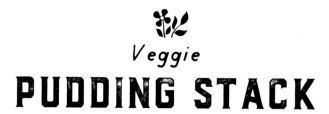

Veggie
PUDDING STACK

One of my weaknesses is white pudding. I love everything about it, from the peppery taste to the texture. I've recently converted to the vegetarian type – still the great taste but with half the calories. Keep your eye out for some of the delicious brands that are now starting to hit the supermarkets. If you can't source vegetarian, this is just as nice made with meat pudding.

SERVES 1

2 baby potatoes, sliced

Low-calorie spray oil

1 decent slice of vegetarian white pudding

3-4 mushrooms, sliced

1 egg

1 60g high-fibre wholemeal bun, halved

1 If not using an airfryer, preheat the oven to 220°C.

2 Pop the potato slices in a microwave bowl with no water and zap them for 5–6 minutes until tender, spray with some oil and pop in the airfryer at 200°C for 10 minutes, or on a tray in the preheated oven for 15 minutes until golden and crisp.

3 Put the pudding slice on some greaseproof paper and using the palm of your hand press it down flat until you have a patty shape. Put a large non-stick pan on a medium heat, spray on some oil and put the patty in one part, then the mushrooms in another, frying off until turning golden. Push these to one side, crack in the egg and cook through.

4 Toast the buns and stack that bad boy up. Layer the bottom bun with the potato slices, then mushrooms, then the pudding patty and finish off with a perfect fried egg. Place the top bun on and give it a little press until the egg breaks and the yolk drizzles down – no sauce needed as this will be just enough.

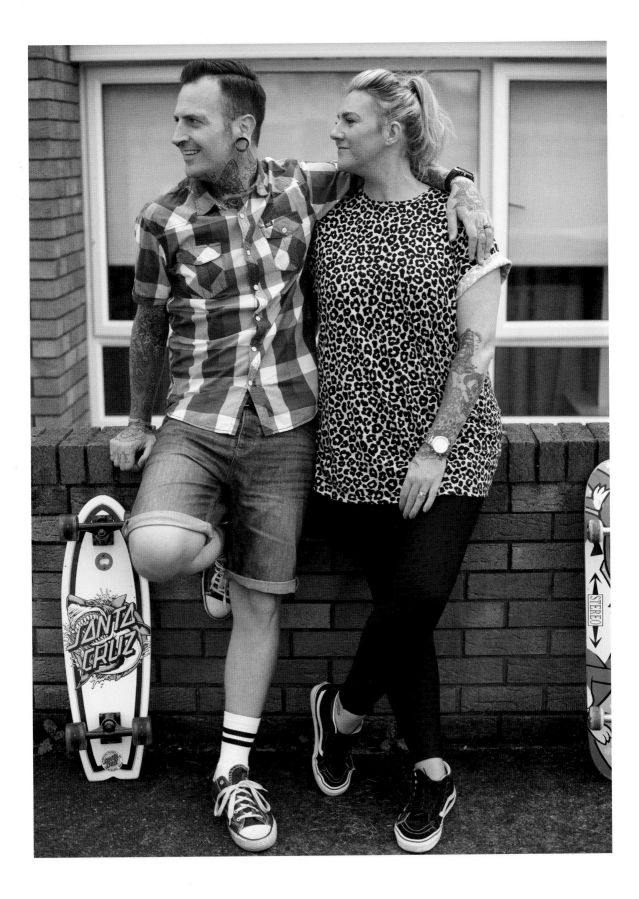

SAUCY
SAUCES

CHEESE SAUCE

Simple, sexy and goes with everything. A great way to jazz up your loaded fries (see Durty Fries, page 149), burgers, actually pretty much anything on your plate. You won't get over how easy it is to make! You'll see this pop up again and again in my recipes – it's so versatile.

SERVES 1

3 light cheese singles, torn
50ml water

1 I get a little pot and pop in my cheese singles and the water. Put the pot over a medium heat on the hob and let the cheese begin to melt and break down. Keep stirring and mixing it with the water. Don't panic if it starts to look a bit scrambled – that's all part of the process.

2 Once it's melted it should become nice and smooth and, depending on your taste, you can add a little extra water to make it more pourable.

Alternative serving suggestion

You can change this up into a rocking nacho cheese sauce by stirring through some chopped jalapeños, 1 teaspoon of hot sauce, and 2 tablespoons of the pickle juice the jalapeños came in.

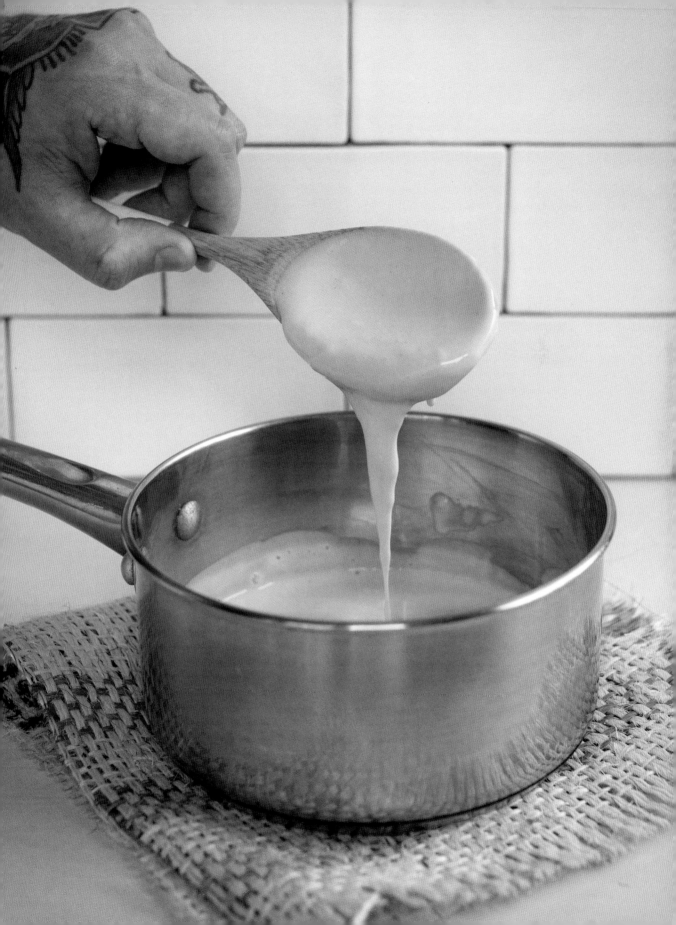

STROGANOFF SAUCE

This is one of my favourite dinners. It's traditionally a Russian dish, but this bad boy was born and bred in County Meath. The flavours of the mustard with the mushrooms is incredible and best of all it takes less than 10 minutes to make. You can serve it as it is with rice or as a sauce for chicken or beef.

SERVES 4

Low-calorie spray oil
2 shallots, finely chopped
3 garlic cloves, crushed
300g mushrooms, sliced
6 light cheese slices, torn
20ml beef stock
1 tsp lemon pepper
1 tsp smoked paprika
1 tsp wholegrain mustard

1 On a hot pan fry off the garlic and shallots in low-calorie spray oil. Add in the mushrooms and fry off until cooked through.

2 Add in the light cheese singles and the beef stock and stir over a medium heat until the cheese melts in.

3 Add in the lemon pepper, smoked paprika and wholegrain mustard. Stir well and bring to a boil, turn down the heat and let simmer for 5 minutes.

4 You should have a nice glossy sauce. If it's too thick, add in a drop of water until you have your desired consistency.

5 Serve with chicken breasts or beef medallions (sautéed separately then sliced) on a bed of wild rice.

GUACAHOLYMOLEY

It was far from guacamole I was raised so never had a taste for it. The first time I tried it I thought it wasn't for me and never revisited it! That was until I started to make it myself and realised I could turn it into something magic with some good seasoning and a pinch of this and a spot of that, so here is my guacaholymoley! You'll see why it's named that after you taste it!

SERVES 4

½ an onion, chopped

6–7 red jalapeños (from a jar)

1 large tomato, finely chopped

1 large ripe avocado

4 garlic cloves, roasted (see page 170)

Juice of 1 lime

2–3 tbsp of the jalapeño juice

Black pepper to taste

1 Put the chopped onion, jalapeños, tomato and avocado and roasted garlic into a blender and give them a good blast.

2 Add in the lime and the jalapeño juices, 1–2 grinds of black pepper and give it another zap, until all the ingredients are blended. I like mine a little chunky so just keep an eye on it and stop blending when you have your desired texture.

3 Serve in a bowl and use as a whopper dip with nachos (see page 95) or to top some homemade tacos.

4 Or just grab a spoon and dig in.

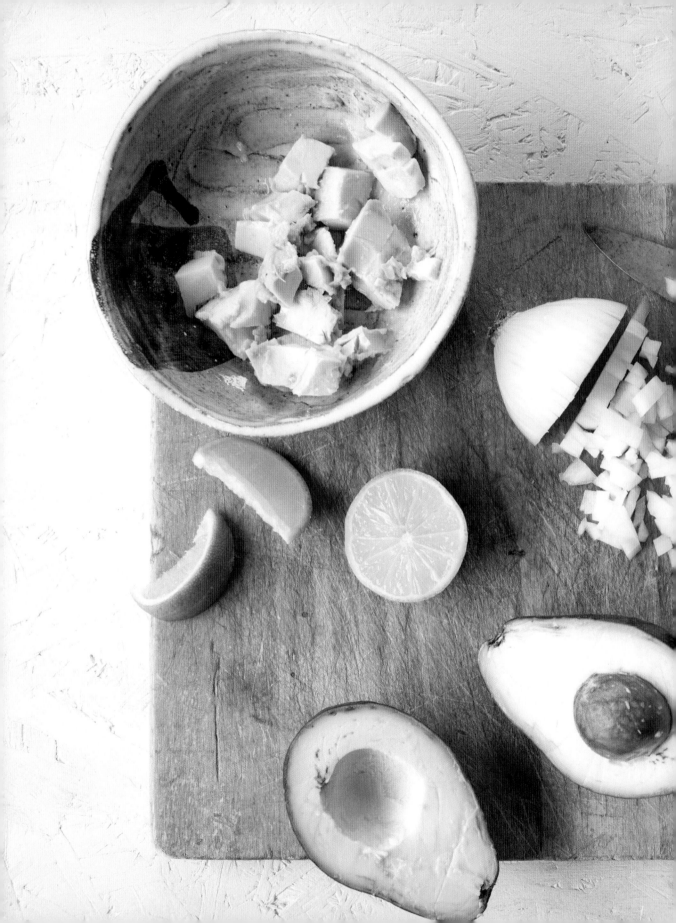

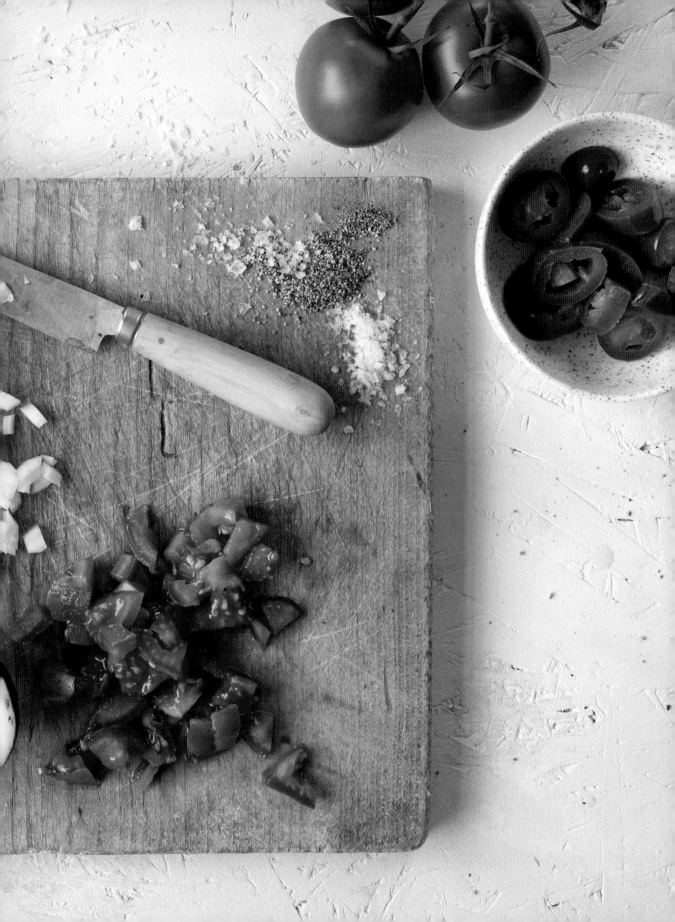

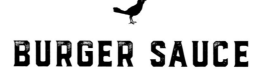

BURGER SAUCE

A burger just isn't a burger without the right sauce. This combination of ingredients will add a little bit of epicness to all your burger creations.

SERVES 1

1 tbsp tomato ketchup

1 tbsp Caesar sauce

1 tsp American yellow mustard

1 pickled gherkin, finely chopped

1 tsp gherkin juice

1 Mix the ketchup, Caesar sauce and mustard together; it should turn a nice peachy colour.

2 Add the gherkin and gherkin juice and stir.

3 Slather over all your epic burgers, absolutely deadly stuff! Store in an airtight jar in the fridge for up to one week.

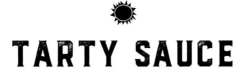

TARTY SAUCE

We made fish and chips one day and had no tartare sauce to go with it – I usually like to have a sauce to accompany my meat or fish – and just like that this little 'tarty sauce' was created. Traditionally tartare sauce has capers in it, but alas I had none so just used what I had to hand in the cupboard.

SERVES 1

1 pickled gherkin, finely chopped

3 tbsp lighter than light mayo

1 tsp yellow American mustard

1 garlic clove, finely minced

Juice of ½ a lime

1 tsp gherkin juice

1 In a small bowl, combine the chopped gherkin with the mayo, mustard and garlic. Mix well to combine.

2 Add the lime and gherkin juices.

3 Taste and see what you think; add more pickle juice if you want more of a bite.

4 Store in an airtight jar in the fridge for up to one week.

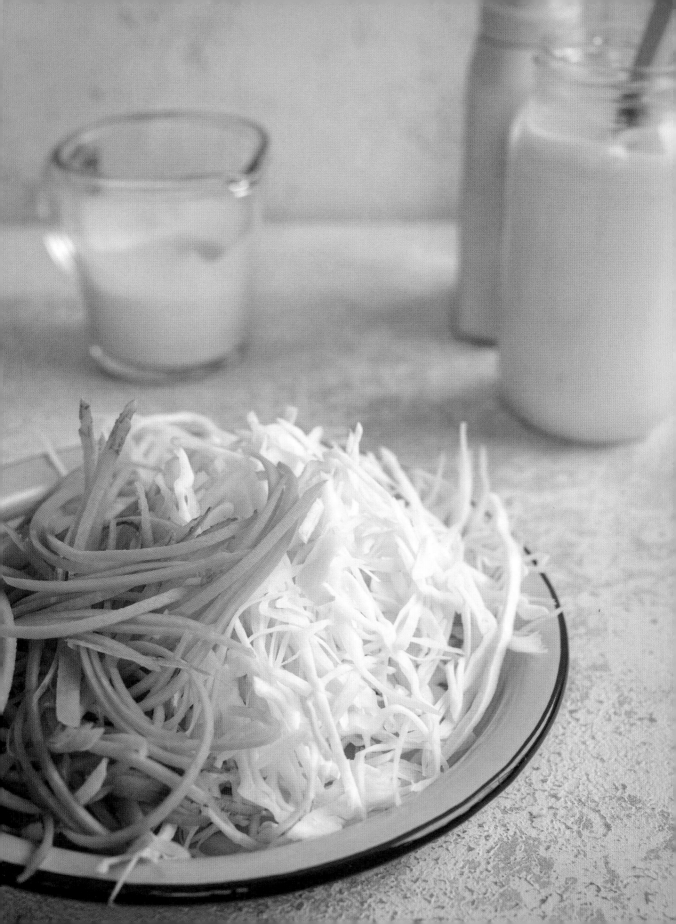

★ ★ ★

Traditional

COLESLAW

Fresh, crunchy and full of goodness, this coleslaw is a perfect accompaniment to a salad or a sambo and fab loaded into a homemade burger.

SERVES 6

½ a white cabbage, finely shredded

2–3 carrots, grated

6 tbsp lighter than light mayonnaise

1 tbsp yellow American mustard

1 tsp apple cider vinegar

½ tsp white pepper

1 Put the shredded veg into a bowl and add the mayonnaise and mustard.

2 Coat the veg evenly with the sauces, then add in the vinegar and pepper and stir well.

3 You can serve immediately, or keep in an airtight container in the fridge for 2–3 days, to be eaten when you fancy a bit of a crunch to go with a meal or a snack.

MISTER DISH'S DISHES

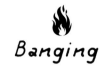

Banging

BLUE BURGER

I'm not gonna lie, burgers are my weakness. You can't bate a big juicy burger, nothing better. My aim here was to come up with an epic, mouth-watering burger that packs a massive flavour punch and won't leave you hungry. The blue cheese is the hero here; it brings everything together and works so well with all the ingredients. Best served with some homemade chips, a cold beer and a hearty appetite.

MAKES 2 BURGERS

500g lean mince

3–4 tbsp panko breadcrumbs

4 heaped tbsp tomato purée

½ tsp cayenne pepper

½ tsp garlic powder

A pinch of salt

A pinch of black pepper

50g blue cheese (such as Cashel Blue)

Low-calorie spray oil

To build the burgers:

2 x 60g wholemeal burger buns, halved

½ a head of lettuce, shredded

1 onion, sliced

2 fresh tomatoes, sliced

1 tbsp burger sauce (see page 140)

1 tbsp garlic mayo

1 Get your mince into a bowl; add in your breadcrumbs, tomato purée, cayenne pepper, garlic powder and a pinch of salt and pepper. Give it a good mix together with your (clean) hands or a fork.

2 Tip the mix onto some greaseproof paper and separate into four equal portions. Using your hands flatten and shape the four portions into burger patties. Take two of the patties and add 25g of blue cheese to each, placing in the middle of the patty.

3 Then take the other two patties (one at a time), and place on top of the cheese-covered patties. Press down around the sides to shape and close them tightly – you don't want the cheese spilling out while cooking.

4 Once both burgers are assembled, get a non-stick pan, lightly spray with oil and put onto a medium heat. Cook burgers on both sides, turning frequently. They should cook in around 15 minutes. Remove to a plate while you get your buns ready. I like to throw them onto the pan for a quick blast to lightly toast them.

5 Put a handful of lettuce on each bottom bun, pop your burger on top, add your onion, tomato, then both sauces and the top bun.

6 Now get ready for the first bite: that flavour explosion. Enjoy.

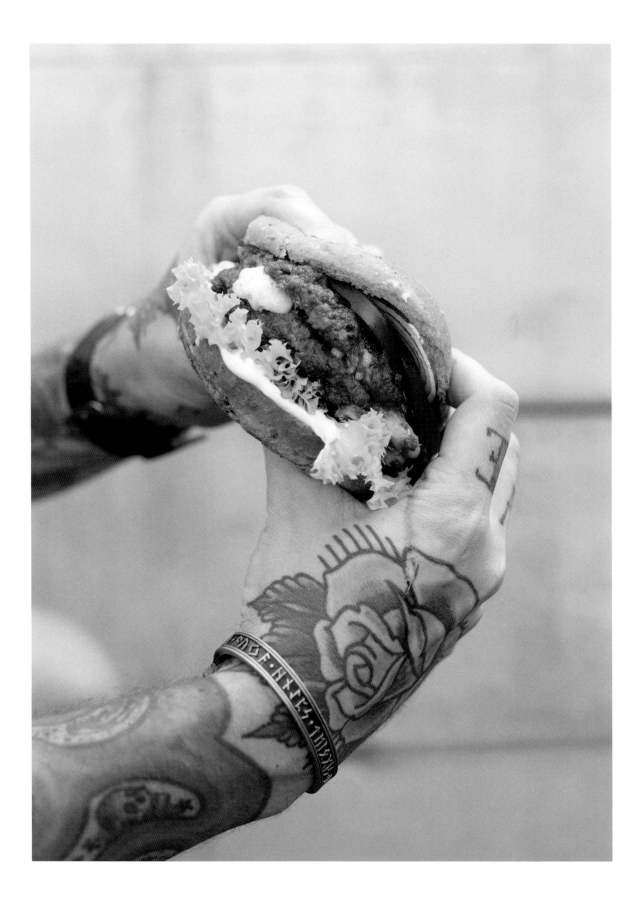

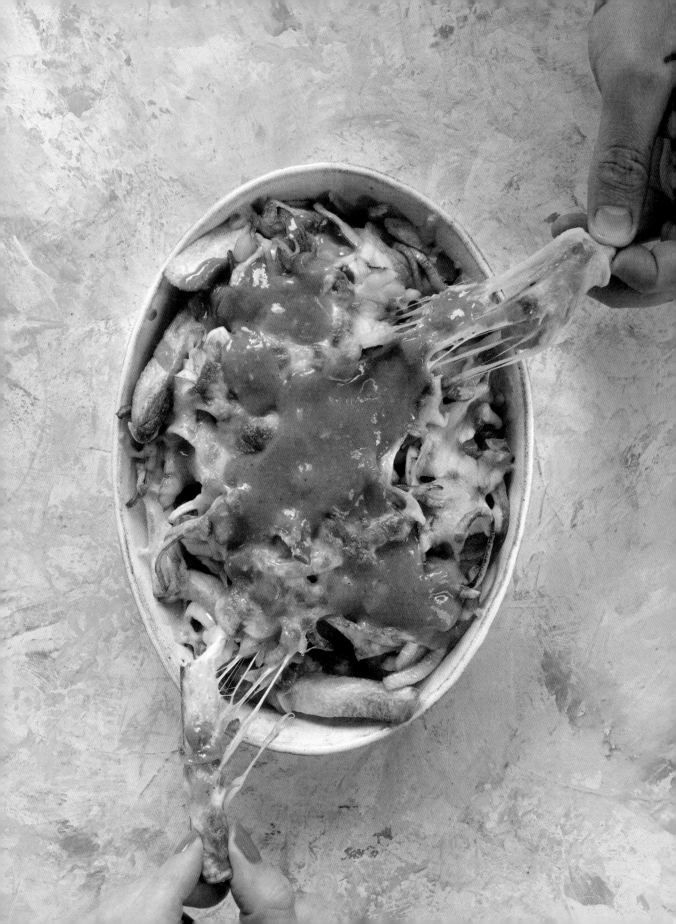

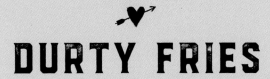

DURTY FRIES

Loaded fries, you cannot and will not go wrong. Gina and myself used to have a thing for garlic and cheese fries, it was our fave treat to get after a night out or if we were getting a takeaway. This is my healthier (and tastier) version. These are epic served alone or as a side, although they are filling enough to satisfy even the heartiest of appetites. Get ready to get durty!

MAKES 2 PORTIONS

2 portions Perfect Chips
(page 44)

Low-calorie spray oil

1 onion, chopped

Salt and pepper to taste

20g jalapeños from a jar

50g mixed grated Cheddar and mozzarella

150ml curry sauce

1 Prepare Gina's Perfect Chips recipe from page 44. While they're cooking, spray a pan with oil and throw your onion on, cooking until translucent.

2 Get your fries, dish up into two bowls and lightly season with salt and pepper. Throw over the onions, jalapeños and cheese, dividing equally between both portions.

3 Place under a medium grill for around 5 minutes to allow the cheese to melt. Once melted, pour your curry sauce over the top and enjoy.

Classic Double
CHEESEBURGER

I remember back in 2007 Gina and myself went to California for a couple of weeks. On that trip I rediscovered my love for the double cheeseburger. I always loved going for the most extreme, biggest burger, but sometimes it's all about going back to basics. There's something special about the double cheeseburger, and my kids love this one as much as I do.

MAKES 2 BURGERS

500g lean mince

2–3 tbsp panko breadcrumbs

2 tbsp tomato purée

½ tsp cayenne pepper

½ tsp garlic powder

Low-calorie spray oil

To build the burgers:

4 light cheese slices

2 x brioche burger buns (or wholemeal if preferred)

4 tbsp burger sauce (see page 140)

½ a head of lettuce, shredded

1 onion, sliced

1 Get your mince into a mixing bowl and add in your panko breadcrumbs, tomato purée, cayenne pepper and garlic powder. Give it a good mix with clean hands, getting everything blended together.

2 Once mixed, pour your mince out onto some greaseproof paper and separate into four equal portions. Using your hands, shape each one into a burger patty.

3 Put a non-stick pan on a medium heat and give a spray or two of oil and then throw your burgers on. Cook for around 15 minutes, turning throughout to ensure they cook evenly. Just as the burgers are ready I like to add the cheese slices while they are still on the pan, allowing them to start melting in.

4 Lightly toast your buns to give them a bit of a crunch, then start to build your burger. Slather burger sauce on the bottom, add the lettuce, two patties, onion and another slather of sauce.

5 There you have it, the classic cheeseburger. Enjoy.

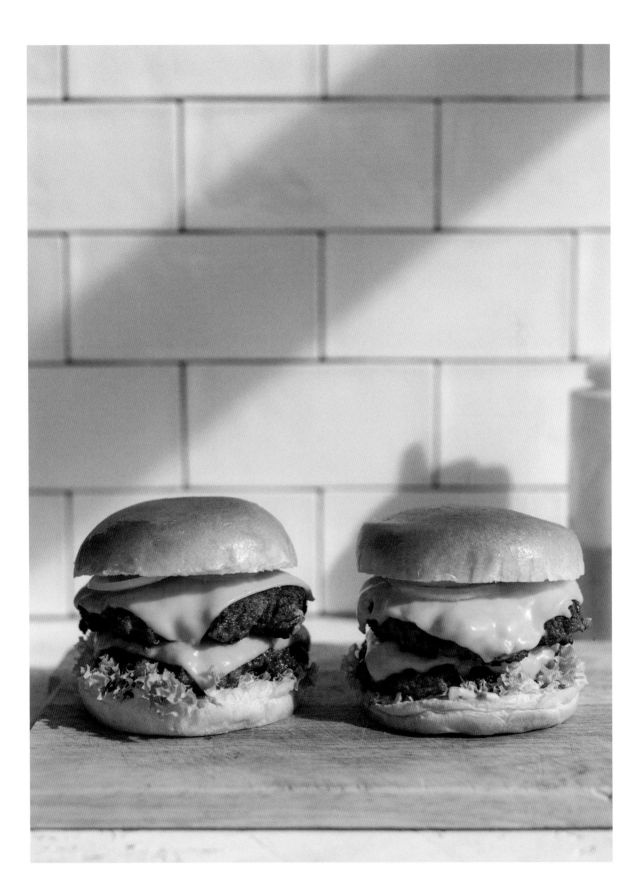

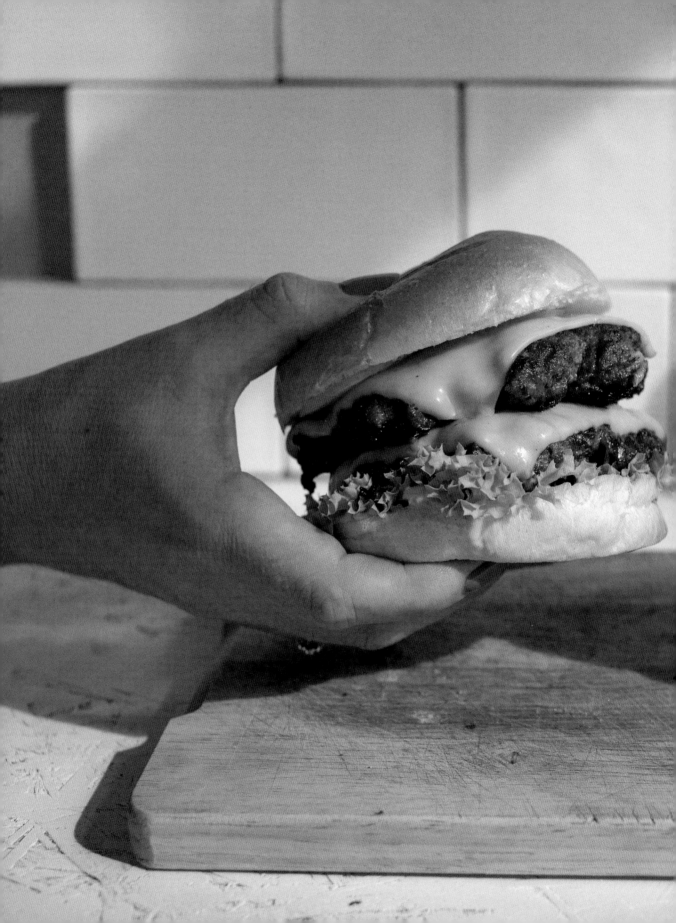

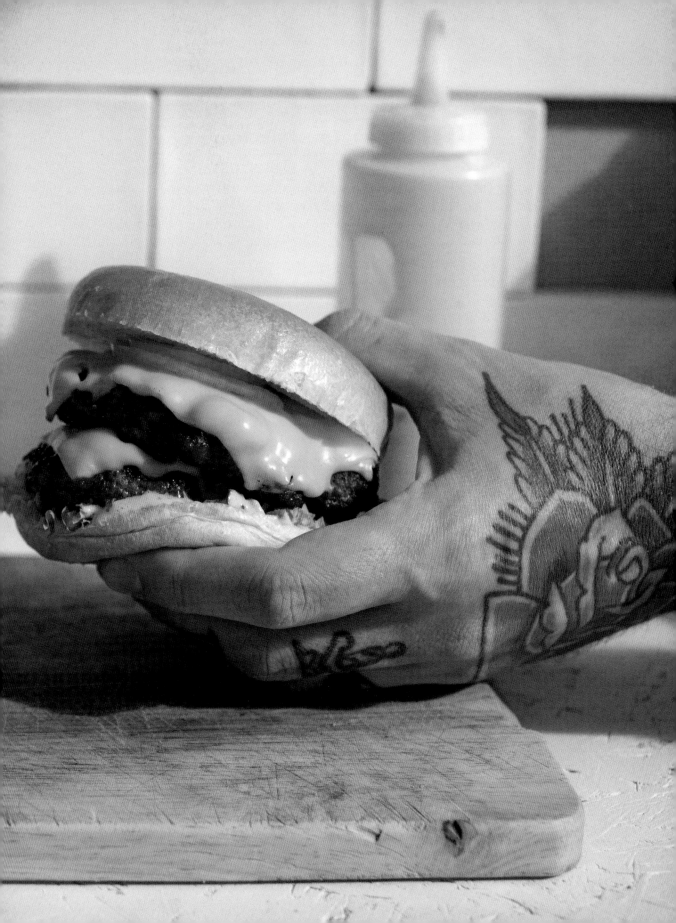

FISH AND CHIPS

As a young teenager I remember walks down by the seaside followed by some takeaway fish and chips for dinner. I loved it, so I wanted to recreate something similar but a lot healthier than the chipper version. In only 30 minutes you'll end up with a banging plate of fish, chips, mushy peas and some homemade dipping sauce.

SERVES 2

2 portions Perfect Chips (see page 44)

1 egg, beaten

20g panko breadcrumbs

1 tsp paprika

1 tsp chilli flakes

1 tbsp lemon pepper

1 tsp garlic powder

2 cod fillets

Low-calorie spray oil

To serve:

1 x 400g tin of mushy peas

Tarty Sauce (see page 141)

1 First off prepare your chips according to Gina's Perfect Chips recipe on page 44.

2 Preheat the oven to 180°C.

3 While your chips are cooking get two bowls. Tip the beaten egg into one and your breadcrumbs, paprika, chilli flakes, lemon pepper and garlic powder into the other. Mix these spices well with the breadcrumbs.

4 One at a time, dip your cod fillets into the egg then into the other bowl, being sure to do both sides to get a good coating.

5 Put both fillets on a baking sheet sprayed with oil in the preheated oven for 12–15 minutes. Turn over halfway through. Your coating should go a nice golden brown colour when cooked.

6 Serve with mushy peas on the side (heated up) and dollops of Gina's Tarty Sauce.

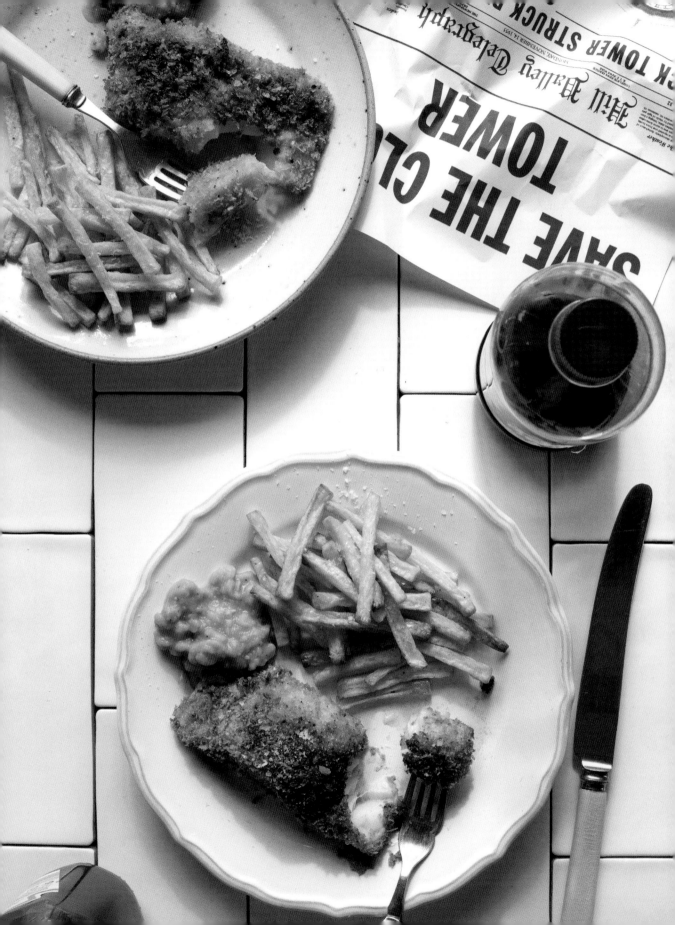

⚓

FISH BURGER

Fancy something different? Well, give this bad boy a try – it's heavy on flavour, light on the waistline, and packs a little kick. Great as a lunch or served with some homemade chips as a main.

MAKES 2 BURGERS

2 large potatoes, washed and peeled

2 spring onions, finely chopped

1 sweet red pepper, deseeded and finely chopped

1 small tin of sweetcorn, drained

1 tbsp lemon pepper

1 tsp cayenne pepper

1 tsp crushed chilli

Salt and pepper to taste

1 x 160g tin of tuna, drained

3 eggs, 1 beaten

20g panko breadcrumbs

Low-calorie spray oil

To build your burgers:

2 x 60g wholemeal burger buns

½ a head of lettuce, shredded

20g low-fat Cheddar cheese

2 tbsp Caesar dressing

2 tsp hot sauce

1 If not using an airfryer, preheat the oven to 180°C.

2 First off, peel and boil those spuds. When they're cooked give them a good mash, add in your spring onions, pepper, sweetcorn, lemon pepper, cayenne pepper, crushed chilli, salt and pepper and your tin of tuna. Time to get stuck in, get those (clean) hands in the bowl and mix up, or use a wooden spoon. Shape into two patties.

3 Get two bowls, and put your beaten egg in one and breadcrumbs in the other. Dip both sides of the fish burgers (one at a time) into first the egg and then the breadcrumbs.

4 Pop the burgers into an airfryer on 180°C for 15 minutes or on a baking tray in the preheated oven for 15–20 minutes. Turn halfway through cooking.

5 Just before your burgers are done, fry up two eggs in a pan, spraying the pan lightly with oil first.

6 Once cooked serve your fish burgers on toasted wholemeal buns topped with the lettuce, Cheddar, Caesar dressing, hot sauce and the fried egg.

7 You can also use the same method for the fish burgers and shape into fish fingers for the kids. These always go down a treat with our two.

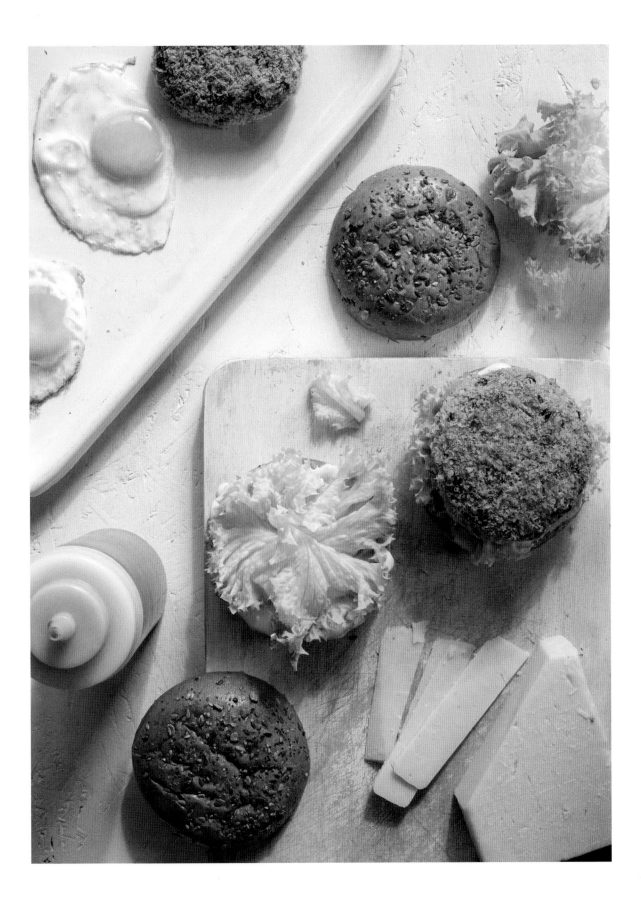

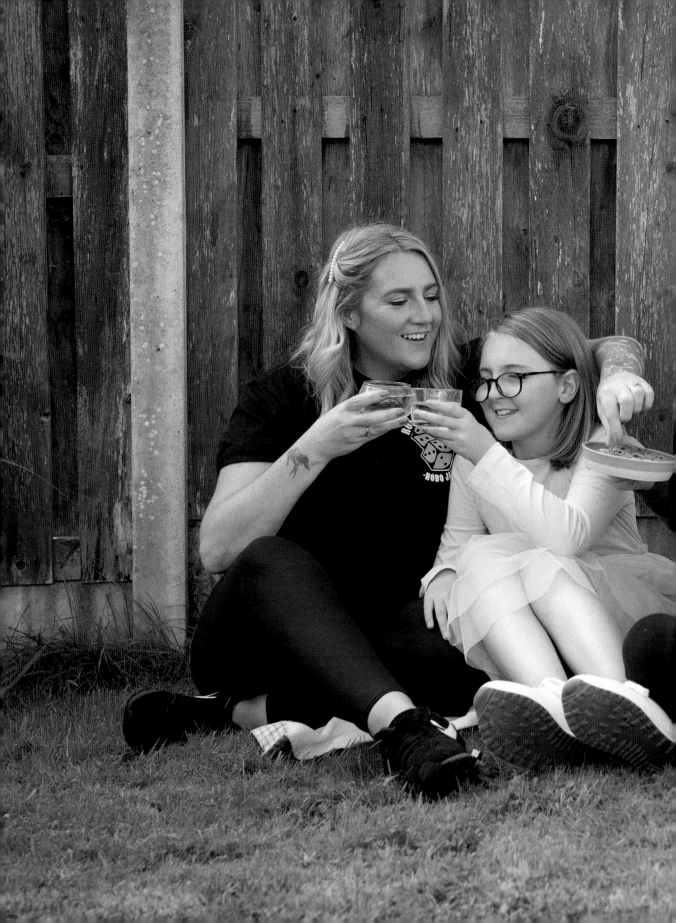

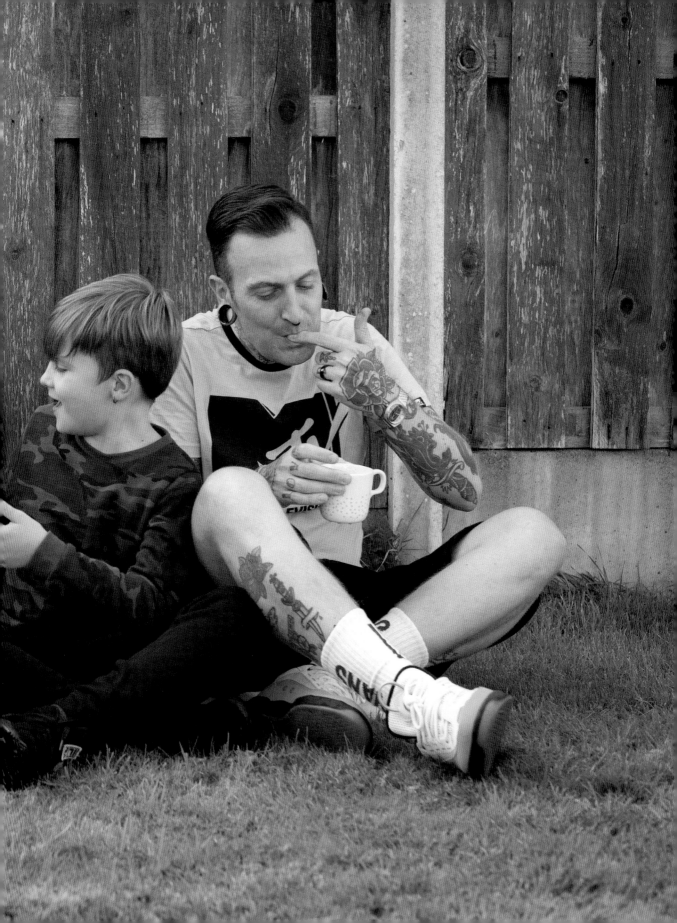

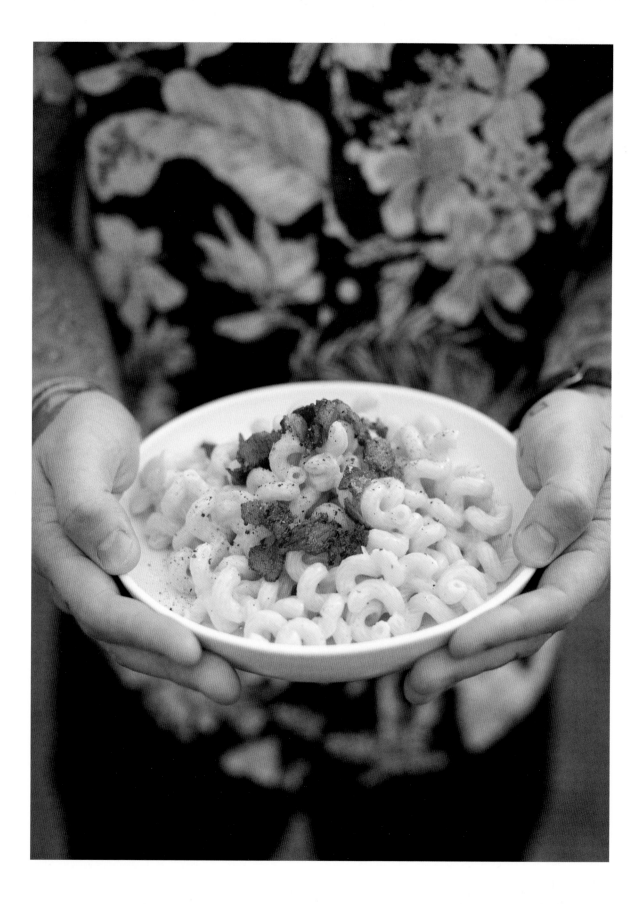

MAC and CHEESE

I made this for the kids one afternoon and they loved it so it's now become a regular staple in the house. Pure simple and pure deadly, proper comfort food. Handy for when the kids come in from school or as a snack/lunch for anybody.

SERVES 2

1–1½ cups pasta (macaroni or penne are good)

3 light cheese single slices, torn

30g low-fat Cheddar

Salt and pepper to taste

1 Get your pasta on, into a big saucepan with boiling water and a pinch of salt and cook for the amount of time it says on the packet.

2 While the pasta is cooking we're going to get the cheese sauce on the go. Grab another saucepan and drop in your cheese slices and Cheddar and add 50ml of water. Pop on a low/medium heat and stir until all melted together.

3 Once your cheese sauce is ready, put to the side and grab your pasta, drain it of all water and throw back into the saucepan. Throw it on a low heat, mix in the cheese sauce and stir well to combine. Add a pinch of salt and pepper to taste.

4 Dish up and enjoy. If you fancy a bit of meat with this, you could sprinkle some crispy bacon over the top.

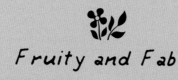

Fruity and Fab

FRENCH TOAST

We've been to the States a few times and one of my fave things when over there is to indulge in some of the awesome breakfasts they have on offer. French toast was always a particular favourite of mine. Sweet or savoury and just downright delicious. This is great for a lazy weekend morning when you want something different. The kids also love this one.

SERVES 2

4 eggs

½ tsp ground cinnamon

1 tsp vanilla extract

4 slices of high-fibre whole-meal bread

Low-calorie spray oil

2–3 tbsp low-sugar strawberry jam

100g strawberries, hulled and chopped

2 kiwis, peeled and chopped

60g blueberries

20g Biscoff biscuit spread (melted in the microwave)

1 Biscoff biscuit

1 Crack your eggs into a mixing bowl, add the ground cinnamon and vanilla extract and whisk thoroughly.

2 Get a non-stick pan on a medium heat and give it a spray or two of oil. Dip your bread into the egg mix on both sides, ensuring full coverage. Then pop onto the pan and cook on each side for 2–3 minutes, until golden.

3 Once cooked grab the first slice of French toast and add a tablespoon of jam, spreading it evenly. Next add half of your chopped strawberries and kiwi (as you're making two portions). Now add the next slice of French toast on top, sprinkle half your blueberries on top, then drizzle half your melted biscuit spread (melt it by giving it a quick blast in the microwave).

4 Break off half of your biscuit and crush, and sprinkle on top. Repeat with the remaining two pieces of bread and serve.

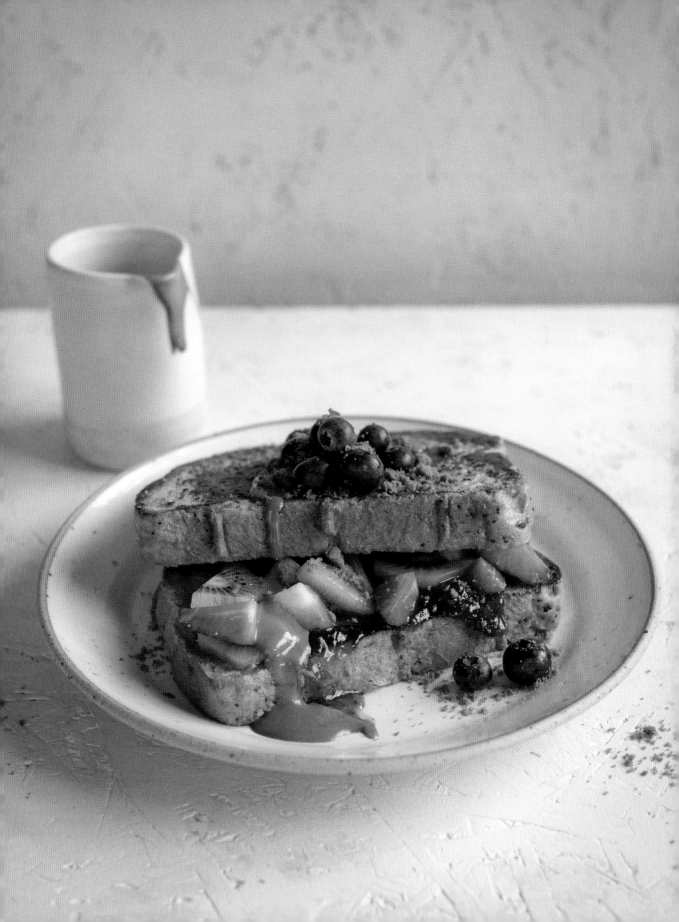

♥

Cheesy Curry
BEANS ON TOAST

Beans on toast, the ultimate comfort food – simple, quick and easy to make. Here's my take on the ultimate classic, it's guaranteed to fill that gap and set those taste buds tingling. Perfect on a cold winter's day to warm you up.

SERVES 2

80g frozen spinach

1 x 400g tin of baked beans

30g mixed grated Cheddar and mozzarella

1 heaped tbsp mild curry powder

4 slices of wholemeal bread

½ tsp chilli flakes

Salt and pepper to taste

1 Defrost your frozen spinach, either in boiling water or in the microwave.

2 While that's on the go, empty your beans into a saucepan.

3 On a medium heat, stir in your cheese and curry powder, mixing thoroughly. Your beans should take on a nice cheesy consistency.

4 Pop your bread in the toaster.

5 Once the beans are cooked grab your spinach, drain it of any water, pop into a bowl and mix in your chilli flakes and a pinch of salt and pepper.

6 Grab your toast and place the spicy spinach evenly on top, then add your beans, some salt and pepper to taste and serve up.

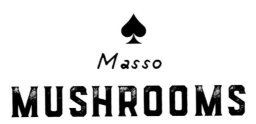

Masso

MUSHROOMS

I absolutely love mushrooms! This is a personal fave of mine to have as a starter on a Friday/Saturday night, although it can be eaten as a snack anytime you fancy something tasty. I've put this recipe together using ingredients that complement each other perfectly and give some banging flavour.

SERVES 2

4 large portobello mushrooms

3 spring onions, finely chopped

1 red pepper, deseeded and finely chopped

6 to 8 hazelnuts, roughly smashed in a pestle and mortar

50g mixed grated light Cheddar and mozzarella

Salt and pepper to taste

Peanut rayu (optional; available in specialist shops)

1 Preheat the oven to 180°C.

2 Line up your mushrooms and divide the spring onion, pepper and hazelnuts between them. Sprinkle over some salt and pepper and top with a generous handful of grated cheese.

3 Pop onto a baking tray and lash into the preheated oven for 15–20 minutes. Plate up and just before serving drizzle a teaspoon of peanut rayu over each one, if you have it.

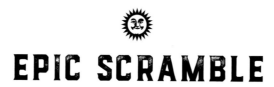

EPIC SCRAMBLE

Who doesn't love scrambled eggs, a cornerstone of many an Irish breakfast and brunch for years? The problem I've always had was I could never find a decent scramble anywhere, so I made it my mission to made an epic scramble that is quick and easy and bursting with flavour.

The first thing to know is that you should never ever cook your scramble in a microwave, never ever! I know it's quick and easy but it doesn't make for a good end result. The method below is super quick, and easy too, and shouldn't take more than 10 minutes.

SERVES 2

1½ tsp lemon pepper

Salt and pepper to taste

5 large eggs

30ml milk

1 tsp butter

1 So, first off get your lemon pepper, salt and pepper and mix all together into a little bowl. Have it on the side ready to rock.

2 Get a small saucepan and crack in your eggs, then add the milk and butter. Put on the hob on a medium heat, get your spatula and stir, stir, stir and stir … don't stop. Not too fast, but keep everything moving about. After 1–2 minutes lift the saucepan up off the heat for 10–15 seconds, continuing to stir. Then pop back onto the hob and repeat. Keep doing this and after a few minutes your eggs will start to scramble.

3 As you stir, drag your spatula across the bottom of the pan to stop the egg sticking.

4 At this point get the bowl of seasoning that you have at the ready, throw it all in and keep stirring.

5 Now, for me, the perfect scrambled eggs should be soft and creamy and not in any way leathery. So as soon as you have a soft, creamy consistency serve up straight away. Perfect on its own on toast or as part of a banging breakfast.

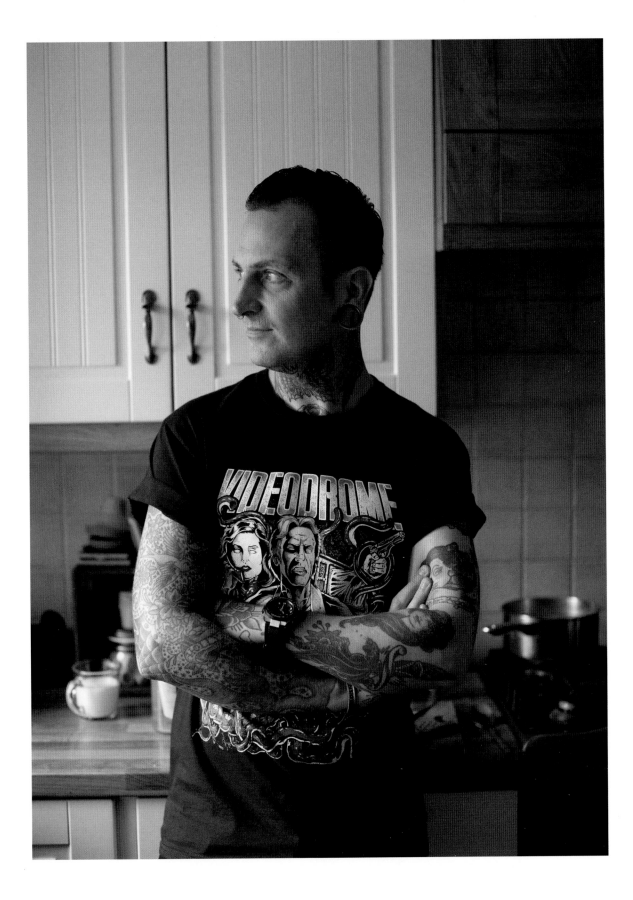

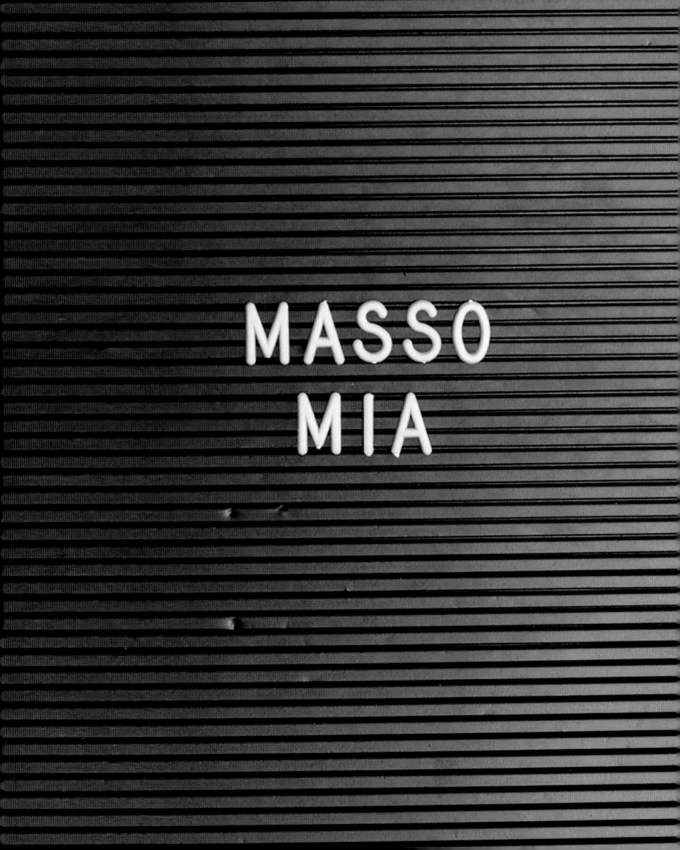

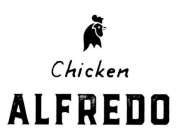

Chicken
ALFREDO

My first time ever trying this dish was on a day trip I took with my friend Grace on a cruise ship. I ordered this for my starter and couldn't stop thinking about it afterwards. As usual, I had to make it the Gina way as soon as I got home. This is a super-simple dish but so rich and creamy and just tastes like more.

SERVES 4

6 cloves of garlic, peeled
Low-calorie spray oil
4 chicken fillets
1 tbsp lemon pepper
300g dried linguine
Salt
400ml chicken stock
150ml light cream
60g Parmesan cheese, grated
Fresh parsley, to garnish

1 If not using an airfryer, preheat the oven to 200°C.

2 First, we are going to roast the garlic. I find it easiest to do this in the airfryer, so I spray the peeled cloves with a little oil and pop them in for 6–7 minutes at 200°C. If you don't have an airfryer, just wrap in foil and place in the preheated oven for 20 minutes until soft. Once ready I squeeze the garlic out of its skins, crush with a pestle and mortar until mushy and leave to one side.

3 For the chicken, remove the scaldy bits, as always. Coat all over with the lemon pepper and pop on a tray in the preheated oven for 25 minutes until golden or in the airfryer for 15-20 minutes at 190°C.

4 To prepare the pasta, boil in plenty of salted water (I use about a tablespoon) according to the pack instructions, stirring occasionally so it doesn't stick to the bottom of the pot, and reduce the heat if it starts to boil over. Drain and keep to one side until the sauce is ready.

5 Now make the sauce. Put the chicken stock, cream, Parmesan cheese and the roasted crushed garlic in a wok or large saucepan (you'll be adding the pasta later) and cook on a medium heat, stirring, for about 10 minutes until blended. The sauce at this stage should be glossy and thick. Tip in your drained pasta and mix to coat every piece in the sauce.

6 Slice or shred your crispy, golden chicken, add it to the pasta and sauce and give it a good stir to coat the chicken in the yumminess of that delicious sauce.

7 Serve in bowls, garnished with some parsley.

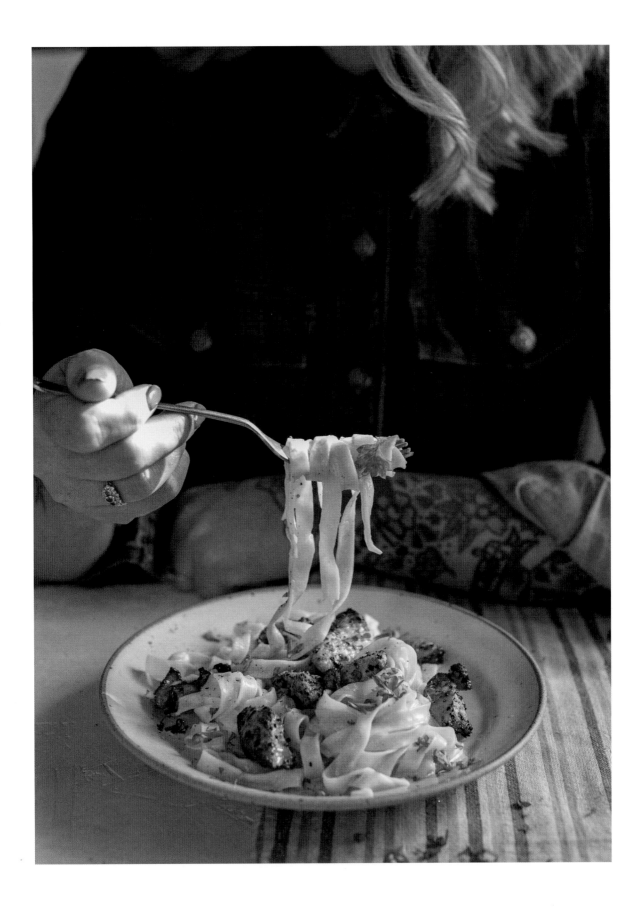

Prosciutto-wrapped
ASPARAGUS

A salty and sweet starter or side dish, oozing with delicious mozzarella. This is perfect when having friends over. Try serving it on wooden boards with herby fries, bruschetta and sundried tomatoes.

SERVES 4 PLUS

12 fresh asparagus spears

12 slices of prosciutto (remove excess fat)

70g light mozzarella, grated

1 If not using an airfryer, preheat the oven to 200°C.

2 These quantities are based on four people having three wraps each but you can increase or decrease the amounts depending on how many you're feeding.

3 Start by parboiling the asparagus for 2–3 minutes until the heavy crunch is gone. Drain and put to one side.

4 Lay out the prosciutto on a board and sprinkle the mozzarella evenly onto the edge of each piece.

5 Take two pieces of asparagus, place directly onto the mozzarella and roll the prosciutto tightly around the asparagus and cheese.

6 Repeat until you have used up all the asparagus and prosciutto, then lay on a baking sheet and cook the rolls in the preheated oven for 10 minutes or until the prosciutto has crisped up. If using an airfryer, pop them in at 180°C for 5–6 minutes.

7 Remove and serve hot. A very impressive nibble!

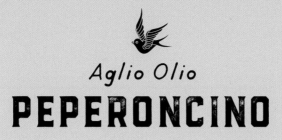

Aglio Olio

PEPERONCINO

Italy is one of our favourite holiday destinations. We love everything about it – the scenery, the people, but especially the food (and the masso wine). This is a super-quick dish with only five easy-to-find ingredients and by the time your pasta is cooked it will be ready to serve. Ideal to keep in the fridge for the lunchbox the next day; heat it up or just lash it into you cold!

SERVES 2

140g dried spaghetti

Salt

2 tablespoons rapeseed oil

2–3 cloves of garlic, crushed

1 fresh red chilli, finely chopped, or 1 tsp chilli flakes

15g Parmesan cheese, grated (more if you love it as much as me)

2–3 twists of the black pepper mill

To serve:

Mixed salad leaves

Fresh tomatoes, sliced

1 Cook the pasta according to the packet instructions in a big pan of boiling water with about a tablespoon of salt (don't worry, the pasta won't absorb all that salt). Give it an occasional stir so it doesn't stick to the bottom of the pot and reduce the heat if it starts to boil over.

2 While the pasta is bubbling away get cracking on the other bits.

3 Put the rapeseed oil in a high-sided pan (I always use me wok) and on a high heat, get it nice and hot then add in the crushed garlic and cook for 2 minutes or until it starts to go brown, making sure you keep it moving so it doesn't stick or burn. Bang in the chilli and let that infuse in the oil for a minute or so.

4 When your pasta is cooked, drain it and pour it into the wok with the oil, garlic and chilli, sprinkle in the Parmesan, give it a good stir, grind over some pepper and plate that baby up!

5 Serve with mixed salad leaves and some fresh sliced tomatoes. Deliziosa aka masso!

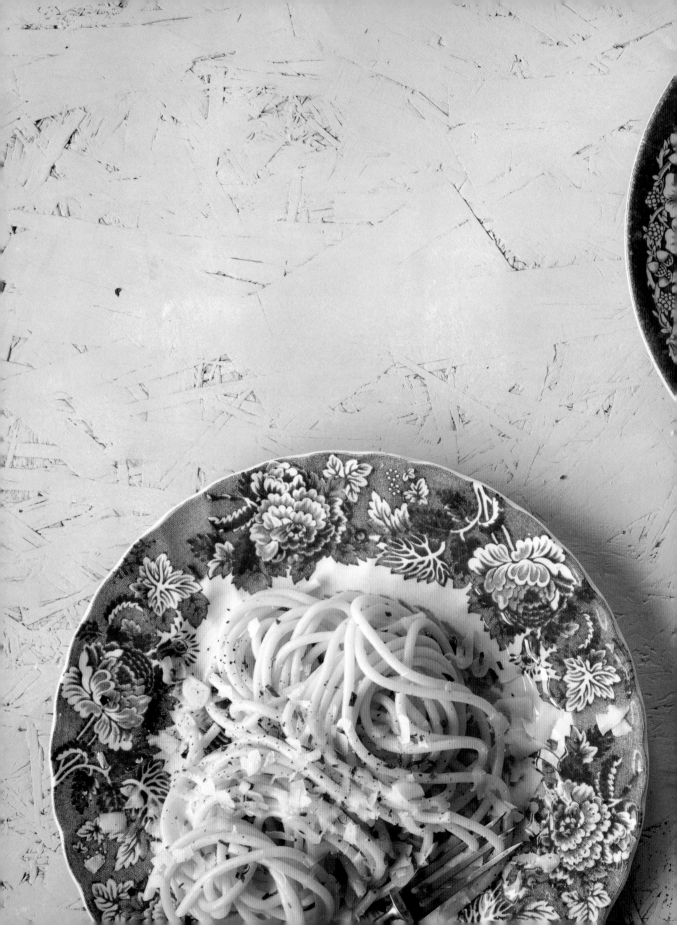

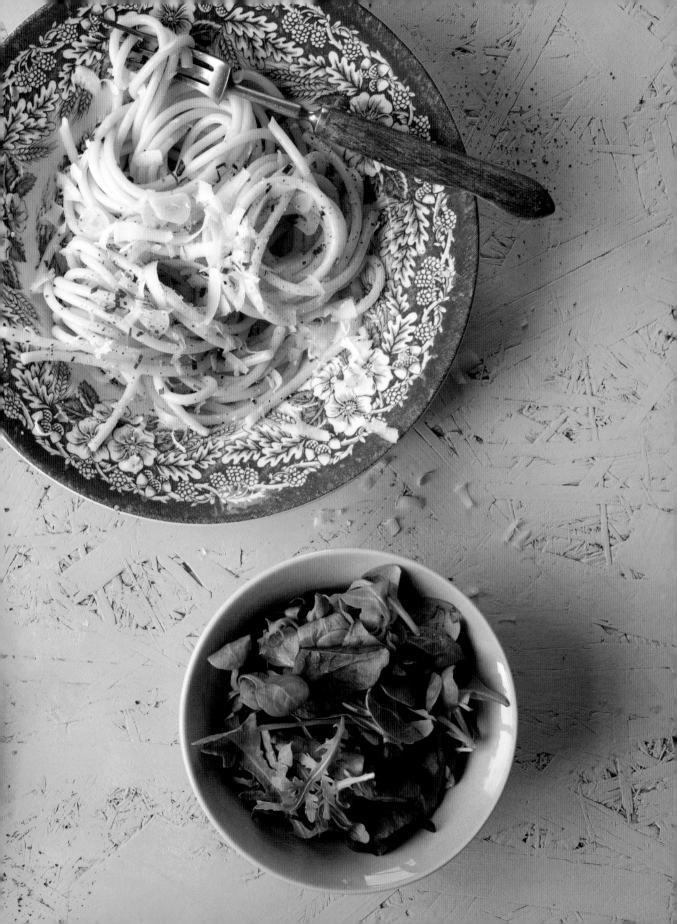

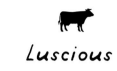

Luscious

LASAGNE

Sometimes you need comfort food, something that just hits the right spot and sends your taste buds to the moon and back. This is a great one for the whole family to enjoy or even make it for yourself and freeze in individual portions to save cooking on another night – score! Goes great with a lovely fresh side salad or even some fab airfryer chips (see page 44). It's MASSO!

SERVES 4

500g lean beef mince

1 tsp garlic powder

1 tsp chilli flakes

1 x 400g tin of chopped tomatoes

½ a 700g jar of garlic passata

1 tsp paprika

1 tsp smoked paprika

1 beef stock pot

1 red wine stock pot

1 tsp soy sauce

5-6 drops Worcestershire sauce

1 tablespoon sweetener (optional)

A 33g sachet of cheese sauce mix

Dried lasagne sheets

70g light mozzarella, grated

1 Put the mince in a hot pan and brown, stirring constantly until it all takes on some colour. Add the garlic powder and chilli flakes (optional, but I like it with a little kick).

2 Next add in the tinned tomatoes and half a jar of passata (you can add more if you like it more saucy), then add the paprika and smoked paprika.

3 Give it a good stir and then lash in your beef and red wine stock pots, let them melt down and give it a good mix. Next throw in the soy and Worcestershire sauce.

4 To take the sharpness out of the tomato base you can add 1 tablespoon of sweetener at this stage. Allow it all to simmer until the sauce starts to thicken.

5 Preheat the oven to 220°C.

6 For the 'white sauce' mix your sachet of cheese sauce (available from most supermarkets) with water in a small pot on a medium heat.

7 Now it's time to get layering. Get a medium-sized baking dish, spoon in half the mince mix, cover with lasagne sheets and then add half the cheese sauce. Repeat so you end up with two layers. Finish off by scattering over the grated mozzarella.

8 Pop into the preheated oven for 35–40 minutes or until golden brown.

9 Take out, cut into four portions and serve up with your choice of accompaniment. Fab.

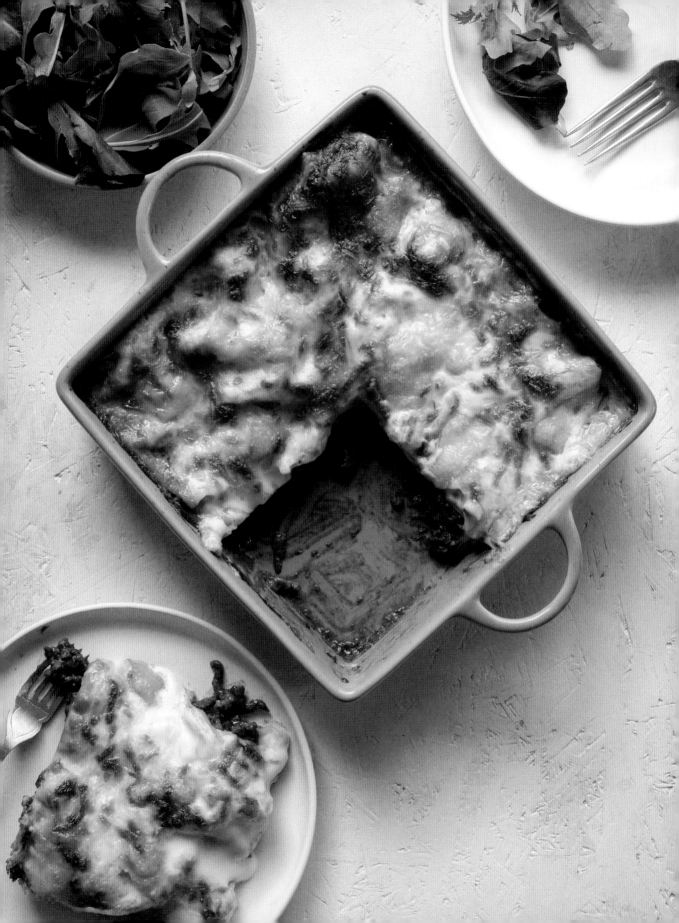

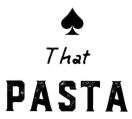

That

PASTA

Rewind to 2006, my Junior Cert home economics practical exam, and this recipe my sister gave me to cook for it. I always remember how beautiful the smell was and I've been making it ever since. It is such a legend, it has become known as 'That Pasta'.

SERVES 4

400g frozen broccoli

Low-calorie spray oil

1 tsp easy/lazy garlic

1 tsp easy/lazy chilli

4 chicken fillets, chopped

1 tsp smoked paprika

350g mushrooms, chopped

250ml chicken stock

45ml light fresh cream

30g low-fat Cheddar cheese

380g dried penne

Parmesan cheese, grated (to serve)

1 Pop the frozen broccoli in some boiling water and into the microwave for 7–8 minutes, drain and leave to one side.

2 Heat a wok or large pan over a medium heat with a few sprays of oil, add in the garlic and chilli and fry off for 2–3 minutes. Add in the chicken and smoked paprika and fry until golden brown.

3 Add in the mushrooms and stir until cooked through, then add in the broccoli.

4 Pour in the chicken stock, cream and cheese and stir over a medium heat until the cheese has melted in. Continue to cook until the sauce begins to thicken and has become nice and glossy.

5 Meanwhile cook the pasta in a large pot of salted boiling water as per packet instructions, then drain.

6 Toss the pasta into the sauce and stir everything through to coat every piece of penne. Serve with a sprinkle of freshly grated Parmesan.

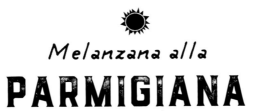

Melanzana alla

PARMIGIANA

This is bit like a lasagne but it uses aubergine layers instead of pasta sheets. We had the pleasure of eating it in a very small traditional restaurant when we visited Rome – the chef even came out to chat to us (in Italian, which we can't speak) and make sure we ate it all. There were lots of ooohhs and aaahhs – a language we can all understand when it comes to food. Gas character!

SERVES 4

2 large aubergines, sliced horizontally into 1cm slices

Low-calorie spray oil

550 ml garlic passata

1 x 400g tin of chopped tomatoes

1 tbsp sweetener

½ tbsp garlic powder

½ tbsp smoked paprika

1 tsp chilli flakes (if you like it spicy)

1 herb stock pot

30g Parmesan cheese, grated

100g light mozzarella, grated

1 Begin by frying off the aubergine slices on a pan with a few sprays of oil until brown. Alternatively you can pop in an airfryer for 6–10 minutes at 220°C until cooked through. When ready, leave to one side.

2 To make the sauce, put the garlic passata, chopped tomatoes, sweetener, spices and stock pot in a large pan over a medium heat.

3 Bring to a boil and stir well until the herb pot has blended into the sauce, then turn down the heat and let simmer for 10 minutes. Now we are ready to build the dish.

4 Preheat the oven to 220°C.

5 In a medium-sized ovenproof dish, spoon in a thin layer of the sauce, a layer of the aubergine so it covers the sauce, then another layer of the sauce with a sprinkle of the Parmesan and some mozzarella. Repeat these layers until you have used up all the aubergine, finishing with a layer of the sauce sprinkled again with the Parmesan and mozzarella (you can also substitute with low-fat Cheddar if you don't have mozzarella).

6 Pop in the preheated oven for 30-35 minutes or until the cheese is melted and golden.

7 Leave it to cool slightly and slice into portions. Serve with a fresh leafy salad or a side of boiled baby potatoes sprinkled with Italian seasoning.

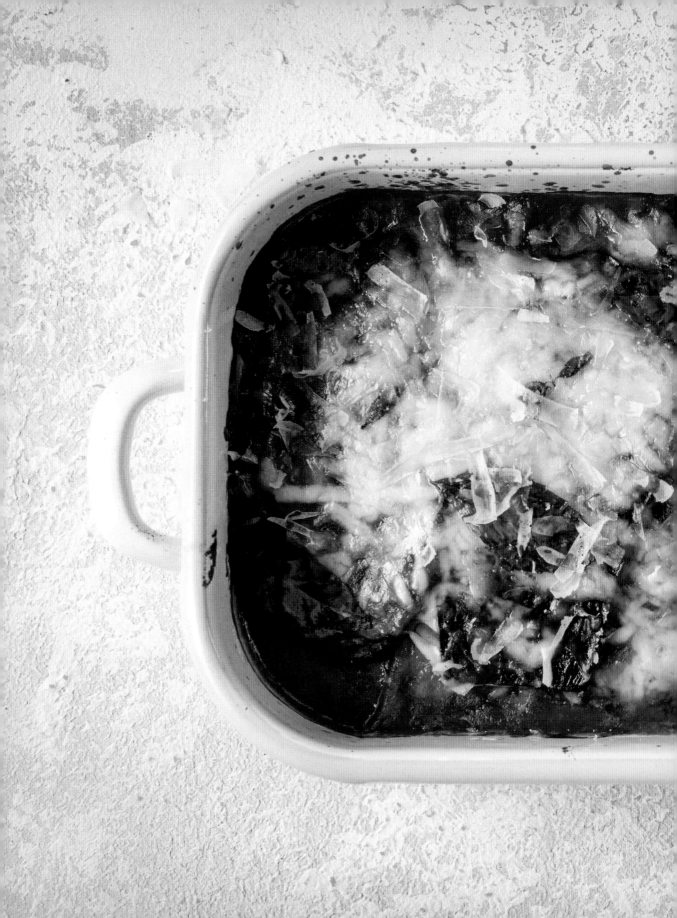

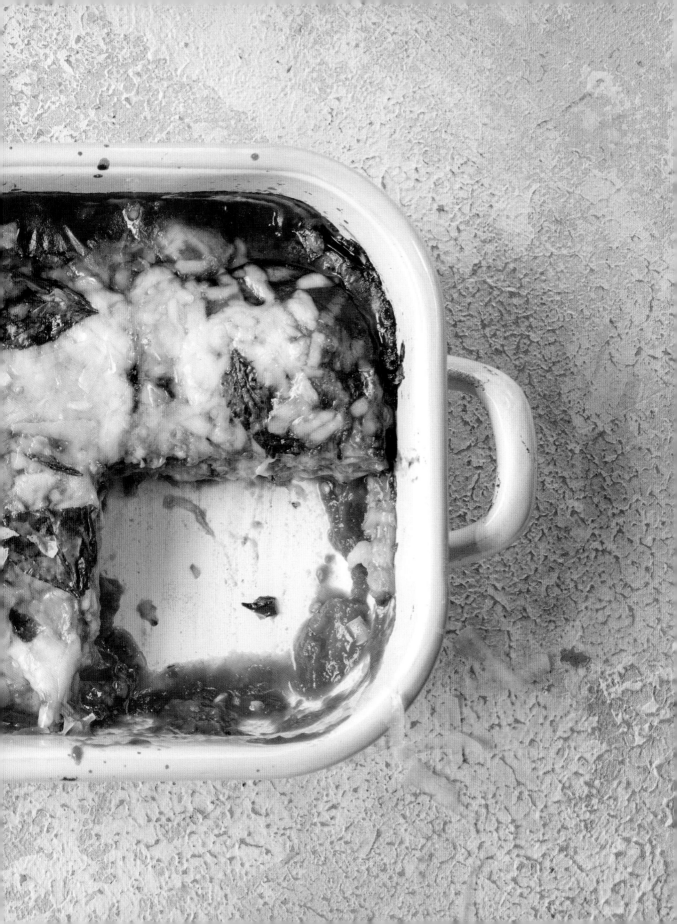

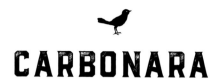

CARBONARA

This old favourite, which needs just a handful of ingredients, couldn't be easier to whip up. When you add the egg yolks to the pasta a kind of magic happens and you get a lovely silky, creamy sauce that is offset by the saltiness of the bacon.

SERVES 4

280 g dried spaghetti

Salt

Low-calorie spray oil

2 garlic cloves, crushed

6 smoked bacon medallions, chopped

3 egg yolks

30g Parmesan cheese, grated (plus extra to serve)

1 Fill a large pan with salted water and bring to the boil, add in the pasta and cook according to the packet instructions.

2 When cooked drain the pasta, keeping aside some of the pasta water.

3 While the pasta is bubbling away, spray a non-stick pan with some low-calorie cooking spray, add in the garlic and bacon and fry off until the bacon has crisped up.

4 In a small bowl, whisk up the egg yolks with the Parmesan.

5 Tip your cooked, drained pasta into the pan and mix well with the bacon and garlic so it soaks up all the lovely juices from the bottom, then remove the pan from the heat.

6 Now pour in the egg mixture and a ladleful of the pasta water. The egg will cook with the heat of the pasta and the pasta water will turn it into a beautifully glossy sauce. Stir through.

7 Serve in bowls with some extra Parmesan to sprinkle over.

★ ★ ★
SPAG BOL

Who doesn't like a spag bol? This massive family favourite can be ready in under 15 minutes. The kids lap this up so that's half the battle. It's also a great way to get a bit of sneaky veg into their little bellies.

SERVES 4

Low-calorie spray oil

500g low-fat beef mince

1 onion, finely diced

700g plain or garlic passata

1 x 400g tin of chopped tomatoes

1 beef stock pot

1 tsp garlic powder

1 tsp smoked paprika

1 tsp paprika

1 tsp mixed herbs

1 tsp sweetener

½ tsp chilli flakes (if you want it spicy)

5–6 drops of Worcestershire sauce

Salt and pepper to taste

300g dried spaghetti

Parmesan cheese, grated (to serve)

1 Start by getting the sauce going. Heat your pan (I use a wok) and spray with some oil. Throw in your mince and brown, then add in the finely diced onion and fry off until translucent.

2 Add in the passata and the chopped tomatoes, give it a good mix with the mince, then add in the rest of your ingredients (not the spaghetti and Parmesan!) and stir well. The beef stock pot will melt into the sauce so there's no need to add water. Bring it to a boil, then turn down the heat and allow to simmer for 10 minutes, stirring occasionally.

3 While that's happening, cook your spaghetti in a large pot of well-salted boiling water for the length of time it says on the packet. Drain and serve in bowls with your sauce ladled over.

4 And that's all, she wrote – all you need is a bit of Parmesan grated over the top and a nice slice of wholemeal bread to mop up the sauce at the end. If bread isn't an option, just lick the plate clean!

Spicy Cheesy
CHICKEN CALZONES

Calzone is made from a pizza base and is stuffed with filling – it's basically a folded-over pizza! Calzones are incredible, but because of the pizza dough they are super-high in calories. In this recipe, I've made a little adjustment and used wholemeal wraps as the 'pizza base', which makes them a tasty, low-calorie dream.

SERVES 4

Low-calorie spray oil

4 chicken fillets, chopped

4 tbsp hot sauce

2 tbsp buffalo hot sauce

350g mushrooms, chopped

10 asparagus spears, chopped

500g baby potatoes cut into chips

6 light cheese singles, torn

4 wholemeal wraps

1 egg mixed with a little water (egg wash)

1 If not using an airfryer, preheat the oven to 220°C.

2 To make the filling, heat up a wok or a large saucepan with 4–5 sprays of oil and brown the chicken. Add in both hot sauces and toss the chicken until coated evenly.

3 When the chicken is cooked, add the mushrooms and asparagus to the pan and cook for 8–10 minutes until softened.

4 Pop the chipped potatoes into a microwave-safe bowl and microwave for 13 minutes. Throw them in the airfryer with a few sprays of oil at 220°C for 20 minutes or pop on a baking tray with a spray of oil and into a preheated oven at 220°C for 20 minutes, until crispy. Turn the oven down to 180°C.

5 Put the torn cheese slices into a pot with 100ml water and stir over a medium heat until the cheese has melted.

6 Tip the chips into the pan with the chicken and veg then pour in the cheese sauce. Give it a good mix until everything is coated evenly.

7 To assemble your calzones, lay out a wrap and spoon 4–5 tablespoons of the filling on one half, then wet the edges and fold the wrap over the top of the filling until you have a semicircle. Press the edges together and pinch with a fork to seal. Brush over some egg wash and give 2–3 sprays of oil. Repeat with the other three wraps.

8 I cook mine in the airfryer for 10 minutes at 180°C or until golden and crisp, but you can oven bake them in the preheated oven for 15–20 minutes. Cut the bad boys in half to serve and watch all that cheesy goodness ooze out.

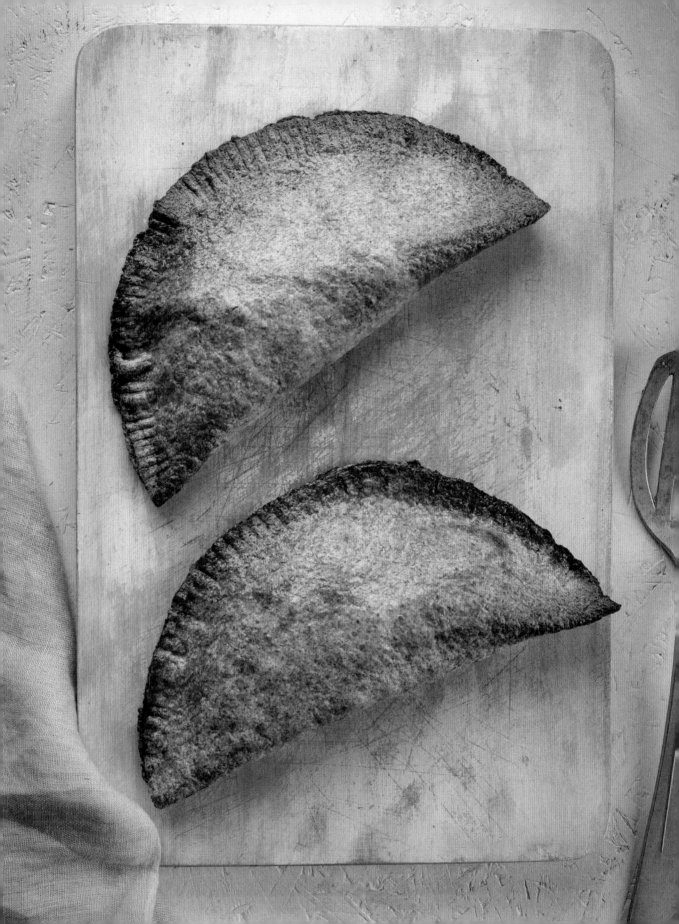

Prosciutto and Mozzarella
PIZZA WRAP

When time is of the essence but the hunger is real, a pizza wrap is the quickest way to curb the belly rumble. I could easily live on these and with the right toppings you have a great Friday night feast that will stop those fingers dialling the takeaway.

SERVES 1

1 wholemeal wrap

2 tbsp BBQ sauce

5 mushrooms, sliced

3 slices of prosciutto

50g light mozzarella, sliced

3 cherry tomatoes, thinly sliced

Low-calorie spray oil

1 Take a wrap and spread on the BBQ sauce right to the edges.

2 Fry off the mushrooms in a pan and scatter over the wrap.

3 Tear up the prosciutto and place it evenly around the wrap.

4 Last, place the slices of mozzarella on top and scatter over the cherry tomatoes.

5 Preheat your grill and spray around the edges of the wrap with oil – this will stop it burning. Pop under the grill for 5–6 minutes until the prosciutto crisps up and the mozzarella begins to melt.

6 When she's ready, place on a chopping board, cut up into slices and eat it while it's piping hot.

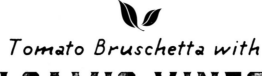

Tomato Bruschetta with
BALSAMIC VINEGAR

For 36 years I've been saying this wrong until my Italian friends told me how to pronounce it the right way. Bruschetta (brews-ke-ta) – scarlet for me! Anyway, bruschetta is a beautiful starter or snack made with crusty toasted bread and topped with something delicious – there are so many different options. I'm going to show you one of my favourites, which is a classic. As you need to marinate the topping, you'll need to start an hour before you want to eat it.

SERVES 4

2 large tomatoes, finely chopped

1 medium onion, finely chopped

1 tsp easy/lazy garlic

1 tsp easy/lazy chilli (optional)

2 tsp balsamic vinegar

5–6 sprays of low-calorie spray oil

15g Parmesan, freshly grated

4 slices of gluten-free sourdough

Salt and black pepper to taste

1 Pop the chopped tomatoes and onion a mixing bowl.

2 Add the garlic, chilli, vinegar, oil and Parmesan, give it all a good mix then cover and refrigerate for an hour to allow all the flavours to mingle.

3 Toast the bread and spoon on the mixture, seasoning to taste with salt and black pepper.

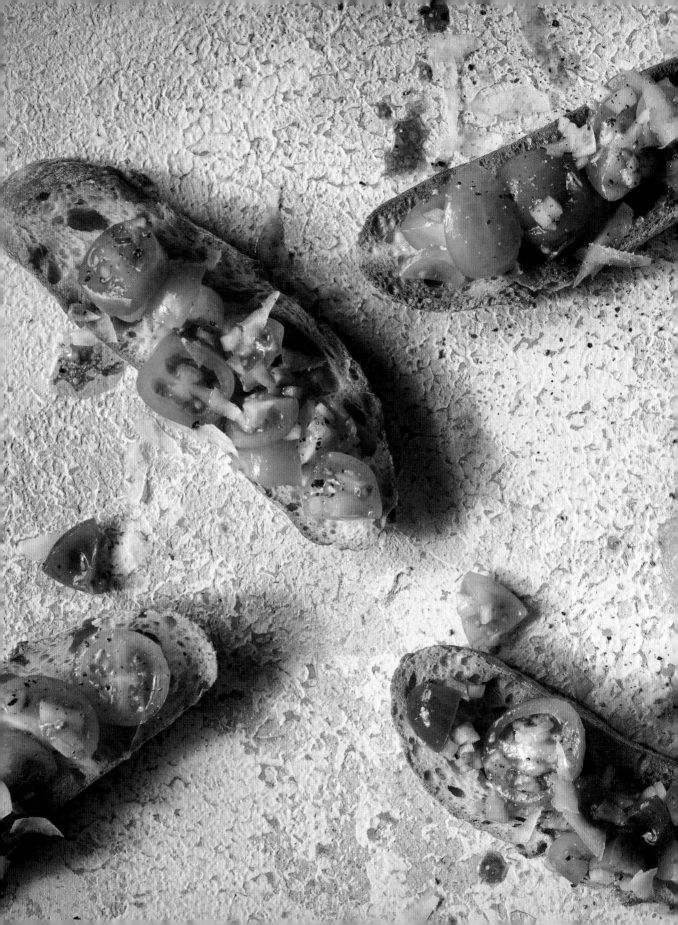

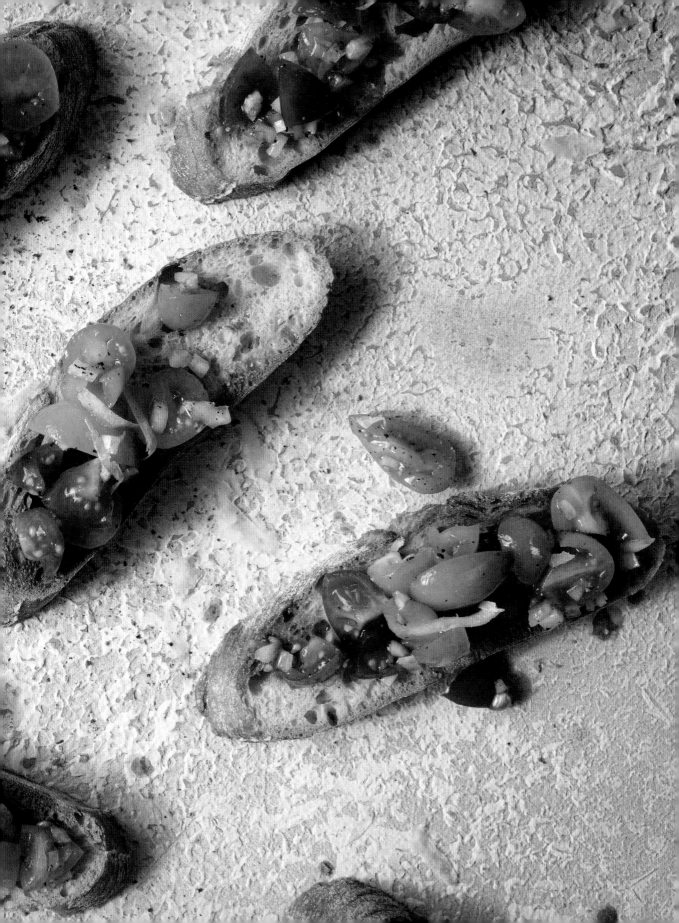

SUPPLI

Suppli, rice balls stuffed with cheese, coated in breadcrumbs and deep fried, are a traditional Italian street food. On a recent trip to Italy we were introduced to these little balls of delight by a small local restaurant we visited each evening for drinks. Although we had no Italian and they had no English we were still able to communicate very well in the language of food. After our first taste we were hooked.

SERVES 6

250g risotto rice

½ medium onion, very finely sliced

200ml passata

½ beef stock cube

1 tsp mixed herbs

½ tsp smoked paprika

4 tbsp frozen petit pois

A pinch of cayenne pepper (optional)

Salt to taste

1 ball of mozzarella, chopped into 6 cubes

2 eggs, beaten

40g panko breadcrumbs

Low-calorie spray oil

1 These work best if the rice is cold, so cook your rice in salted water until al dente and leave to cool.

2 If not using an airfryer, preheat the oven to 200°C.

3 Fry off the onion in a large pan until translucent, then mix in the passata, ½ beef stock cube, herbs, smoked paprika and petit pois, bring to the boil and allow to simmer for 2–3 minutes. Remove from heat and let cool.

4 Add the cooked rice to the sauce and mix well until combined. If you like a little kick you can add in a pinch of cayenne pepper at this stage. Add some salt to taste.

5 Wet your hands, which must be clean. Making sure the mix is cool, take a palm-sized piece of the rice mix, flatten out into your palm and pop in a cube of mozzarella.

6 Fold the rice around the cheese to form a croquette shape and lay out on greaseproof paper.

7 Repeat until you have used up all your rice mixture.

8 Put the beaten egg in one bowl and the breadcrumbs in another, then carefully dip each croquette in the egg, followed by the breadcrumbs.

9 Pop on a baking tray with a spray of oil and bake in the preheated oven for 20–25 minutes until golden and crisp, turning halfway through. You can also put them in an airfryer for 15 minutes at 180°C with a spray of oil.

10 Remove and allow to cool for 1–2 minutes, then tear them open and watch the fabulous mozzarella ooze from the inside.

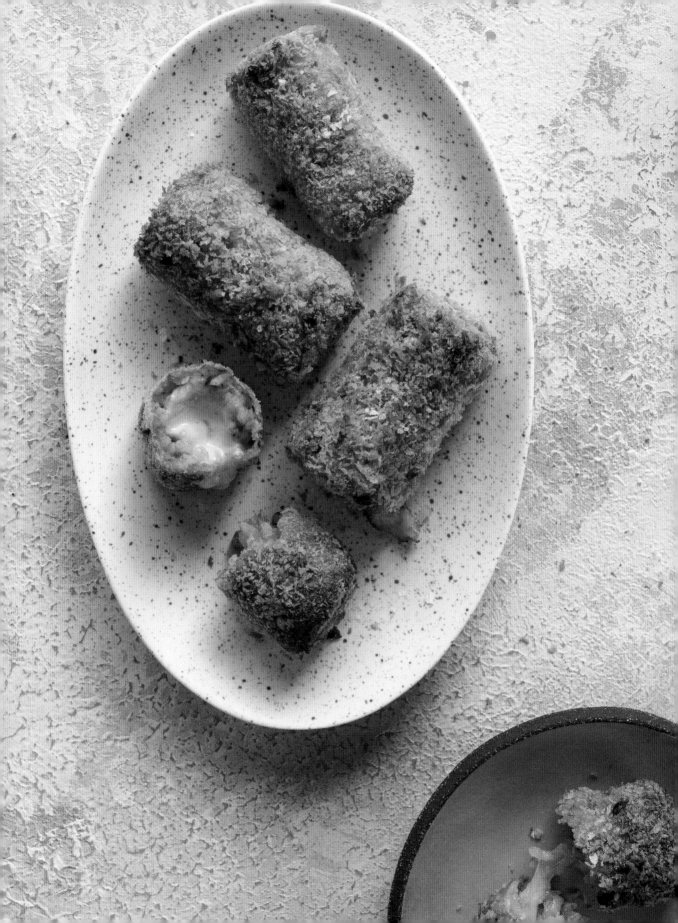

DEADLY & DELICIOUS

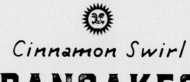

Cinnamon Swirl

PANCAKES

There's one word for these babies and it's MASSO! We cannot get enough of them in our gaff, the kids look for them every weekend, and I love making them. You can jazz them up with different toppings but if you know me then you'll know Biscoff is my life and I find it very hard to cheat on it with anything else. When ya know, ya just know!

SERVES 1

For the batter:

40g porridge oats

2 eggs

50ml skimmed milk

2 tsp sweetener

½ tsp baking powder

½ tsp ground cinnamon

Low-calorie spray oil

For the topping:

1 tsp brown sugar

½ tsp ground cinnamon

2 tsp Biscoff biscuit spread, melted

1 Biscoff biscuit, crushed

1 For the pancakes, put all the ingredients (apart from the oil) into a blender and blitz until you have a nice smooth mixture. Spray a hot pan with some oil and pour in a thin layer of the pancake batter until it covers the entire bottom of the pan. Turn the heat down to medium – you don't want the pancake to burn.

2 Wait 2–3 minutes for bubbles to appear and the top is firming up then flip it over to cook the other side. When it's golden brown on both sides remove and place on a wire rack.

3 Repeat until all the mixture is used up – you should get 2–3 pancakes out of it.

4 When you have all your pancakes cooked, lay them out on a board and get on with your topping.

5 Mix the brown sugar and cinnamon together, then wet your hand with some water and run it over the top of the pancakes – this will allow the sugar and cinnamon to stick.

6 Sprinkle the sugar mix over the top of each pancake and pat it down with your hand.

7 Roll up each pancake into a Swiss roll shape, cut into 5cm slices and assemble in a mug or small bowl.

8 Drizzle the Biscoff spread over each portion, then finish by crumbling the biscuit over the top. Dig in while they're piping hot.

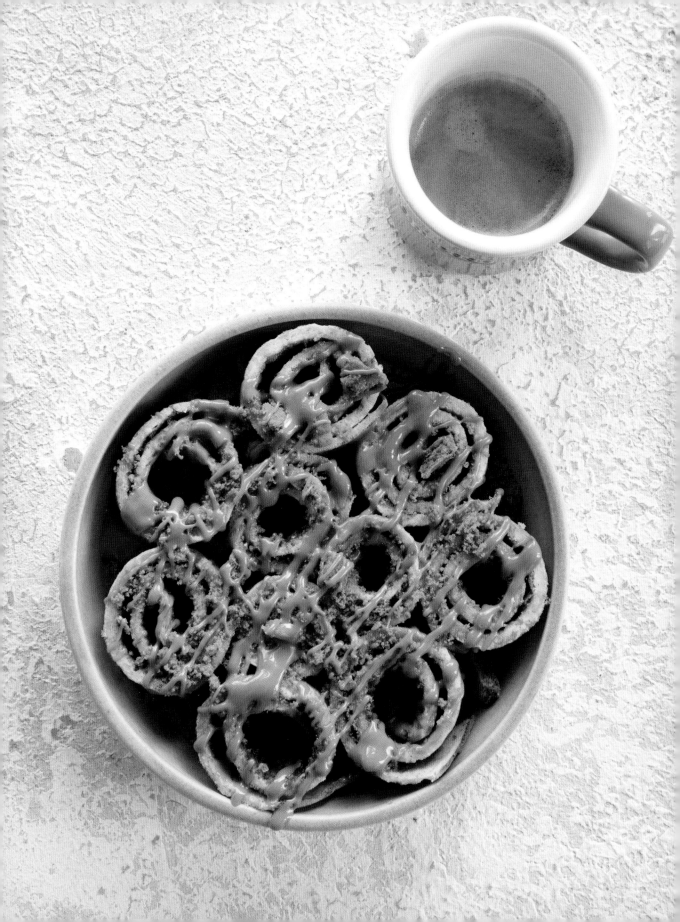

Red Velvet
BREAKFAST PANCAKES

Breakfast is the most important meal of the day so it's only right you should treat yourself to these slimming-friendly red velvet pancakes in the morning. Besides looking amazing, they pack a punch to the taste buds, are super easy to make and the kids love them.

SERVES 1

For the batter:

2 eggs

40g porridge oats

50ml skimmed milk

4 drops of vanilla extract

4–5 drops of red food colouring

2 tsp cocoa powder

¼ tsp ground cinnamon

1 tbsp sweetener

½ tsp baking powder

Low-calorie spray oil

For the topping:

Fat-free vanilla Greek yoghurt

Fresh berries

Shop-bought low-calorie chocolate sauce

1 Put all the ingredients for the batter (apart from the oil) into a blender and blitz until you have a nice smooth mixture.

2 Spray a hot pan with some oil and pour in about a palm-sized amount of the mixture. Reduce the heat to medium and wait until the top is covered in tiny little holes before flipping over. Repeat with the rest of the batter – you should get about five pancakes from the mix.

3 Once cooked, layer up the pancakes in a stack with vanilla Greek yoghurt in between each one, top with berries and drizzle over some low-calorie chocolate sauce.

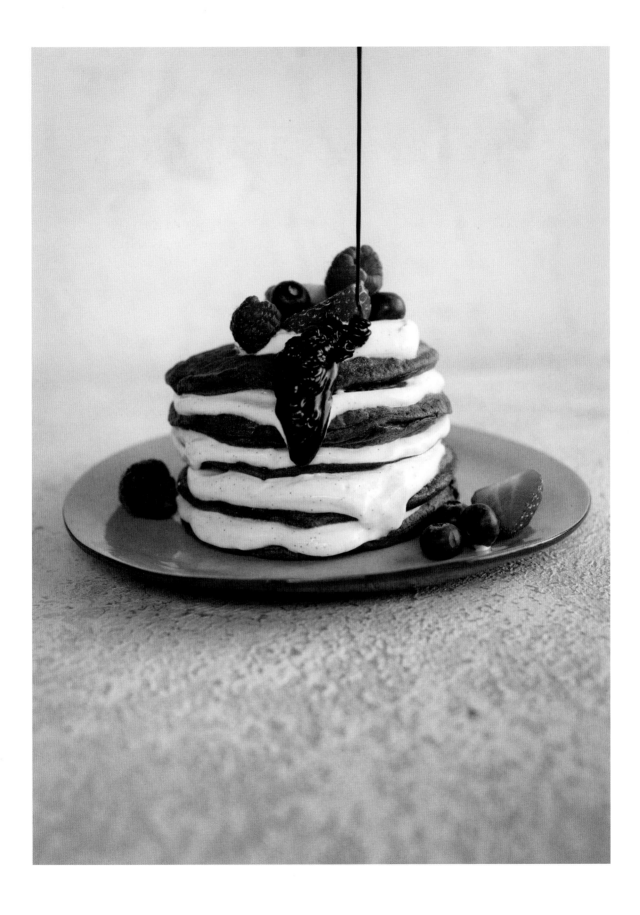

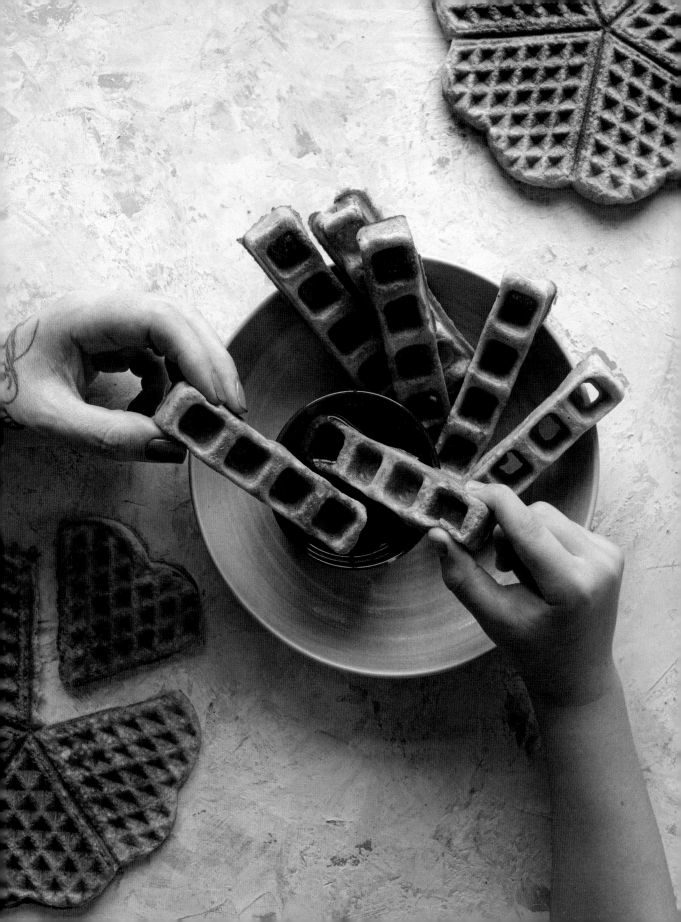

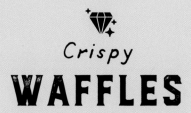

Crispy WAFFLES

No matter what time of the day it is, it's always a good time for waffles! These oat waffles are quick and easy to make and can be dressed up with the toppings of your choice. You'll need a waffle maker or mould to make them.

SERVES 4

80g porridge oats

100ml skimmed milk

1 tsp baking powder

4 eggs

3 tbsp sweetener or zero-calorie syrup

½ tsp ground cinnamon

Low-calorie spray oil

1 Put the oats, milk, baking powder, eggs, sweetener and cinnamon in a blender and give it a good blitz until you have a smooth batter.

2 Preheat your waffle iron and give it a light spray with the oil. Pour in the mixture up to the lip – be careful not overfill as it will overflow out of the sides when you close the lid.

3 Leave for 6–7 minutes until the mixture is cooked through and the outside is crisp. All appliances will vary so just keep an eye on the waffles.

4 Remove the first batch and repeat until the mixture is used up (you'll have quite a lot of batter so you'll be making a few batches). It's a good idea to warm the oven to about 160°C so you can keep the cooked waffles warm while you make the rest.

5 We love to serve ours with super-crispy smoked bacon bits and a cheeky drizzle of maple syrup! Divine.

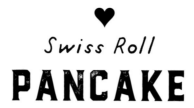

Swiss Roll
PANCAKE

This is a gorgeous little sweet treat that can be made in minutes and eaten at any time of the day. Ideal to kick-start your morning or to enjoy sliced up with a nice strong coffee mid-morning.

SERVES I

For the batter:

2 eggs

40g porridge oats

40ml skimmed milk

4 drops of vanilla extract

2 tsp cocoa powder

½ tsp ground cinnamon

1 tbsp sweetener

½ tsp baking powder

Low-calorie spray oil

For the topping:

100g fat-free vanilla Greek yoghurt

Fresh berries

Honey or maple syrup (optional)

1 Put all ingredients for the batter (apart from the oil) into a blender and blitz until you have a nice smooth mixture.

2 Spray a hot pan with some oil and pour in all the batter. Keep on a medium heat to allow the pancake to cook through without burning. Once the bubbles start to appear and the top becomes solid, gently flip over and cook the other side for 2–3 minutes.

3 Remove from the heat and allow to cool for 5–10 minutes on a wire rack.

4 To serve the pancake, spread over the Greek yoghurt and roll it up. Pop it on a plate seam-side down and slice in half. Sprinkle over the fresh berries and drizzle over a syrup of your choice.

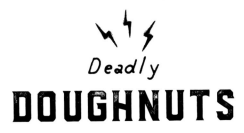

Deadly
DOUGHNUTS

These are perfect snacks you can enjoy with a nice cup of tea or grab and go if you are on the run. You get your sweet hit and they will keep you full until dinner. Get creative and add the toppings you love and even get the kids involved to create some yummy school snacks. You'll need a doughnut maker or mould to make these bad boys.

SERVES 2

For the batter:

40g porridge oats

100ml skimmed milk

½ tsp baking powder

½ tsp ground cinnamon

2 eggs

1 tbsp sweetener or zero-calorie syrup

Low-calorie spray oil

For the topping:

20g Biscoff biscuit spread

1 Biscoff biscuit or hundreds and thousands sprinkles

1 Put all the batter ingredients (apart from the oil) in a blender and give it a good blitz until you have a smooth mixture.

2 Preheat your doughnut maker and give it a light spray with the oil.

3 Pour the mixture into the holes in the doughnut maker up to the lip – be careful not overfill as it will overflow out of the sides when you close the lid.

4 Leave for 6–7 minutes until the doughnuts are cooked through and the outsides are crisp. All appliances will vary so just keep an eye on the doughnuts. Remove and leave to cool on a wire rack.

5 Melt the biscuit spread for about 20 seconds in the microwave in a large ramekin (big enough to dip the doughnuts in) and crush up the biscuit into crumbs.

6 Dip the top of each doughnut into the spread and then sprinkle over the crushed biscuit or the hundreds and thousands.

7 These look so awesome when they are finished, you might want to eat them all at once ... but hey, that's okay!

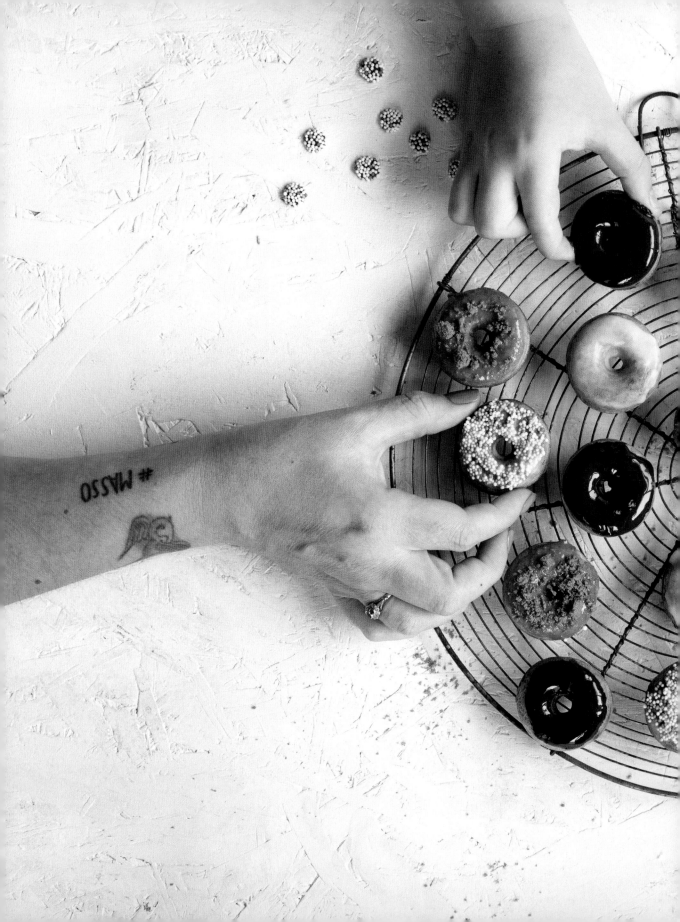

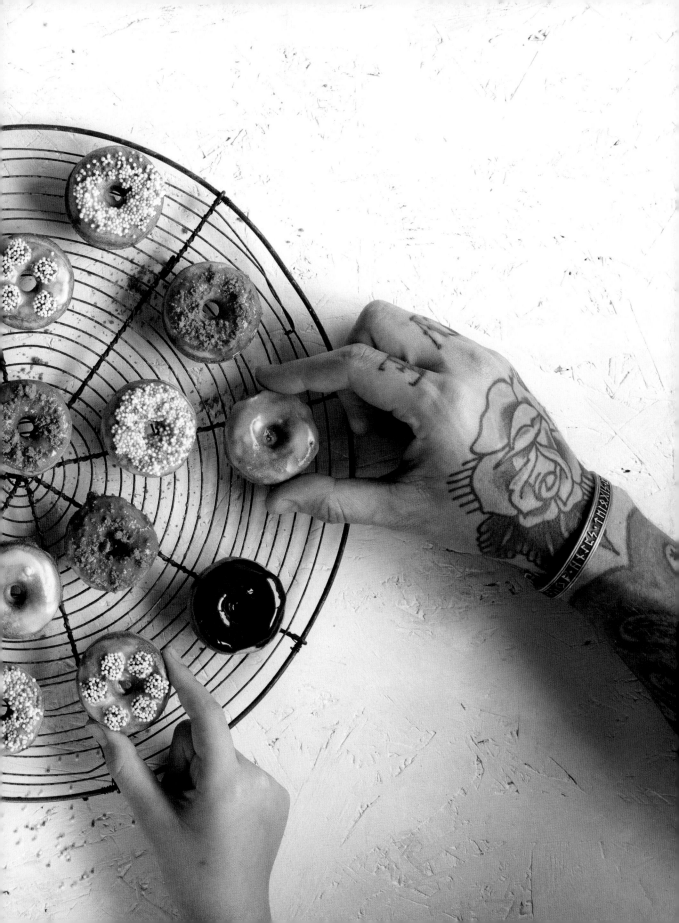

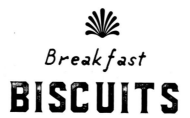

Breakfast
BISCUITS

In the past I used to skip breakfast, which was not a good idea – come lunchtime I'd be so hungry I'd reach for the convenience snacks, and then it would be all downhill from there. These biscuits are perfect to make the night before and keep in an airtight container so you can grab them in the morning when you're running out the door and be full until lunchtime.

MAKES 6 BISCUITS

40g porridge oats
2 tsp light butter, melted
1 egg
1 tsp sweetener
½ tsp ground cinnamon
½ tsp baking powder
4–5 drops of vanilla extract
Low-calorie spray oil

1 Preheat the oven to 200°C.
2 Mix all the ingredients (except the oil) in a bowl until everything is well blended.
3 Spray a baking tray with some oil and spoon out six portions of the mixture. Flatten down with the back of the spoon until you have a cookie shape.
4 Bake in the preheated oven for 15–20 minutes until golden brown, then remove and place on a wire rack to cool. You can jazz these up with some chocolate chips, adding them into the bowl at the mixing stage.

♣

CAKE IN A CUP

When you need a little something a little bit of cake will sort you right out! Now you can have your cake and eat it too – in three minutes!

SERVES 1

40g porridge oats

1 egg

½ tsp baking powder

50ml skimmed milk

3–4 drops of vanilla extract

1 tbsp of sweetener

To serve:

Light squirty cream

Fresh berries

Biscoff biscuit spread, melted

1 Put the oats in a medium-sized microwave-safe mug.

2 Add the rest of the ingredients and give it a good stir, making sure the egg is completely mixed through.

3 Pop in the microwave on a high setting for 3 minutes. During this time it should rise up nice and high and have a spongy texture when you touch the top. If it is still a bit wet, pop it back in for another 30 seconds.

4 You can dig in and eat it straight from the cup or turn it out onto a plate and add some cream and fresh berries, or if you want it to be whopper, drizzle some melted biscuit spread over the top. Get it into ya!

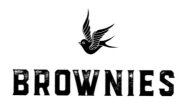

BROWNIES

Little bites of chocolatey goodness, these are great for a sweet snack or a dessert treat.

SERVES 2

40g porridge oats

2 eggs

2 tsp dark cocoa powder

½ tsp baking powder

50ml skimmed milk/water

3–4 drops of vanilla extract

1 tbsp sweetener or zero-calorie syrup

15g carrots, grated (optional)

To serve:

Low-fat yoghurt

Fresh berries

1 Preheat the oven to 200°C.

2 Put all the ingredients, apart from the optional carrots, into a blender and blitz until you have a smooth batter. If using, add in the grated carrot now and give a quick blitz to keep it chunky for texture.

3 Divide the mixture between four ramekins and pop in the preheated oven for 20 minutes.

4 After 20 minutes, stick a knife into the middle of one – if it comes out clean, they are ready.

5 Leave to cool and serve topped with fresh berries and your favourite low-fat yoghurt.

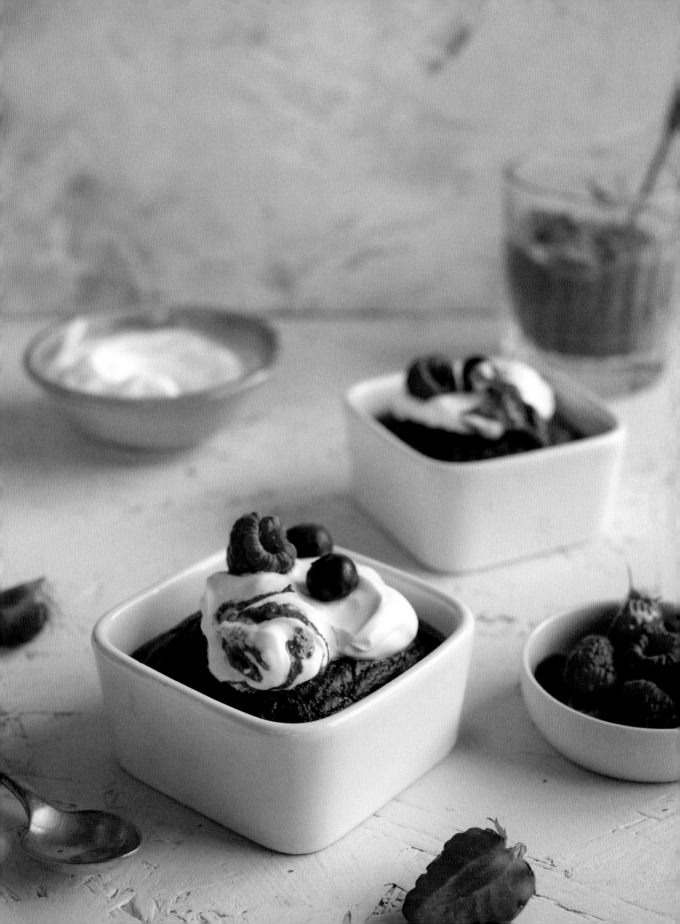

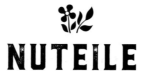

NUTEILE

Hazelnuts, chocolate ... What's not to love? This is a lovely little recipe that the kids can join in and help with. Perfect spread on toast or simply as a dip with breadsticks.

MAKES MANY PORTIONS

2 tsp dark cocoa powder

12 hazelnuts

20g porridge oats

1 tsp rapeseed oil

2–3 drops of vanilla extract

1 tbsp sweetener

A splash of water

1 Put all the ingredients in a blender and blitz it like nobody's business until it's as smooth as you can get it.

2 Have a little taste and see if you need to add more sweetener.

3 Pop it into a small jar and keep it in the press – ideal for the kids for school. They'll never know the difference.

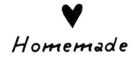

Homemade

BISCOFF SPREAD

Okay, so this is a little treat that can be kept in a jar and used to spread on rice cakes, dolloped onto your porridge, slathered over some homemade pancakes ... the list goes on. Biscoff is a traditional spiced biscuit from Belgium and is usually served with coffee in cafés. I am slightly obsessed with this little golden beauty so I have made my own homemade version of the spread.

SERVES LOADS

1 pack of Biscoff biscuits

1 tbsp rapeseed oil

Not even joking ... That's all you need.

1 Put the biscuits and the oil into a blender.

2 Blitz the Jaysus out of it until it is super smooth.

3 Grab a spoon, lash it into it and taste the wonder that is Biscoff spread.

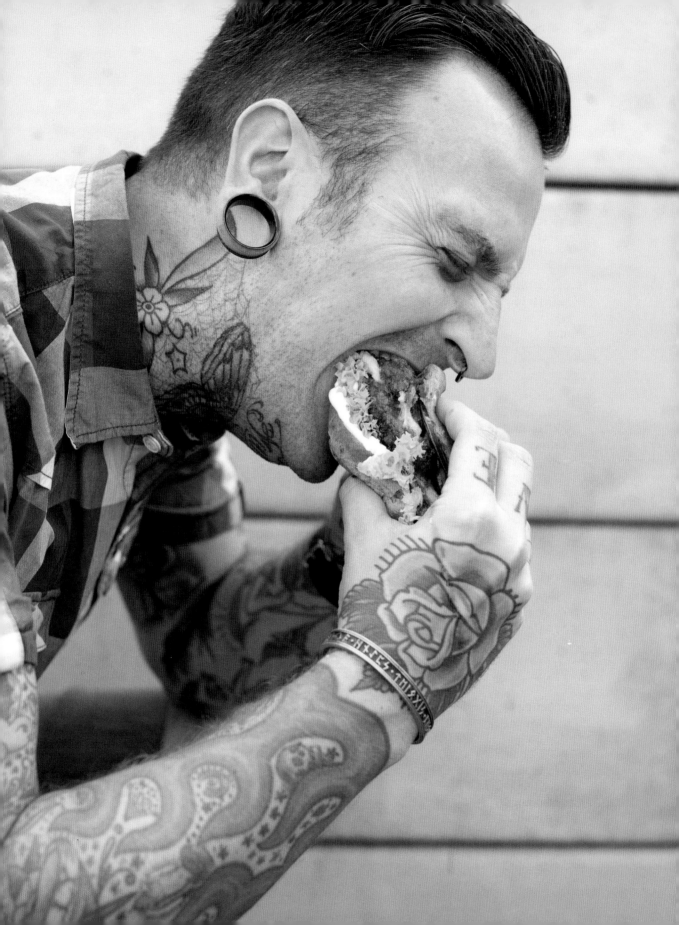

INDEX

A

Aglio Olio Peperoncino 173
airfryers 4–5
    Airfryer Chicken 47
    Airfryer Frickles 50
    Airfryer Omelette 58
    Airfryer Pizza Bagels 56
    Honey and Sriracha-glazed
        Airfryer Brussels Sprouts
        52
asparagus
    Airfryer Omelette 58
    Mushroom and Asparagus
        Soup 124
    Prosciutto-wrapped
        Asparagus 172
    Spicy Cheesy Chicken
        Calzones 184
    Super-speedy Spring Rolls
        76–7
aubergines, Melanzana alla
  Parmigiana 179
avocado, Guacaholymoley 137

B

bacon
    Bubble and Squeak 40
    Carbonara 182
    see also ham; pork
Banging Blue Burger 146
bean sprouts, Teriyaki Yuk
  Sung 74
beans
    Beef Burrito 30
    Cheesy Curry Beans on
        Toast 164
beef
    Banging Blue Burger 146
    Beef and Stout Stew 24
    Beef Bulgogi 28
    Beef Burrito 30
    Classic Double
        Cheeseburger 150

Cottage Pie 33
Daly Dog, The 111
Doner Kebab 83
Luscious Lasagne 176
Mexican Chilli Bowl 25
Not Szechuan Beef 84
Philly Cheese Steak 22
Spag Bol 183
Teriyaki Yuk Sung 74
Terrifically Tasty Beef
    Satay 10
berries
    Brownies 206
    Cake in a Cup 205
    Fruity and Fab French
        Toast 162
    Red Velvet Breakfast
        Pancakes 196
    Swiss Roll Pancake 200
Best Southern Fried Chicken,
  The 48
Biscoff biscuits/spread
    Cinnamon Swirl Pancakes
        194
    Deadly Doughnuts 201
    Fruity and Fab French
        Toast 162
    Homemade Biscoff Spread
        209
Black Bean Crispy Chicken 73
Breakfast Biscuits 204
broccoli, That Pasta 178
Brownies 206
brussels sprouts
    Bubble and Squeak 40
    Honey and Sriracha-glazed
        Airfryer Brussels Sprouts
        52
Bubble and Squeak 40
Buffalo Fries 80
Buffalo Veggie Wrap 94
Burger Sauce 140

burgers
    Banging Blue Burger 146
    Classic Double
        Cheeseburger 150
    Fish Burger 156
    Vegan Burgers 38

C

cabbage
    Bubble and Squeak 40
    Doner Kebab 83
    Traditional Coleslaw 143
Cake in a Cup 205
Carbonara 182
carrots
    Beef and Stout Stew 24
    Brownies 206
    Cottage Pie 33
    Doner Kebab 83
    Sexy Spice Bag 63–4
    Super-speedy Spring Rolls
        76–7
    Traditional Coleslaw 143
    Vegan Burgers 38
    Veggie Fingers/Nuggets 53
cauliflower, Vegan Burgers 38
cheese
    Airfryer Omelette 58
    Airfryer Pizza Bagels 56
    Banging Blue Burger 146
    Beef Burrito 30
    Buffalo Fries 80
    Buffalo Veggie Wrap 94
    Cheese Sauce 134
    Cheesy Chickrizo Pasta 18
    Chicken Enchiladas 14
    Chicken, Leek and Chorizo
        Pie 13
    Chickpea Waffles 120
    Cinema-style Nachos 95
    Classic Double
        Cheeseburger 150

Daly Dog, The 111
Durty Fries 149
Fish Burger 156
Garlic and Cheese Fries 65
Mac and Cheese 161
Masso Mushrooms 165
New Yorker, The 107
On-the-pan Cheese Toastie 106
Philly Cheese Steak 22
Rockin' Reuben Salad 119
Sausage and Egg Muffin From Scratch 101
Spice Bag Burger 70-2
Sticky Chicken Burger 89
Stroganoff Sauce 136
That Pasta 178
see also mozzarella; Parmesan cheese
Cheese and Onion Crisps 114
Cheesy Chickrizo Pasta 18
Cheesy Curry Beans on Toast 164
chicken
Airfryer Chicken 47
Best Southern Fried Chicken, The 48
Black Bean Crispy Chicken 73
Buffalo Fries 80
Cheesy Chickrizo Pasta 18
Chicken Alfredo 170
Chicken and Leek Vol-au-Vents 23
Chicken Enchiladas 14
Chicken Fried Rice 86
Chicken Kiev 36
Chicken, Leek and Chorizo Pie 13
Crispy Chicken Fillet Roll 98
Crispy Tikka Chicken Kebabs 90
Faddyjattys 34
Katsu Curry 21
Me Ma's Chicken Curry 16
Sexy Spice Bag 63-4
Spice Bag Burger 70-2

Spicy Cheesy Chicken Calzones 184
Sticky Chicken Burger 89
Sweet and Sour Chicken 68
That Pasta 178
chickpeas
Chickpea Waffles 120
Not Nuts Nuts 115
Vegan Burgers 38
chorizo
Cheesy Chickrizo Pasta 18
Chicken, Leek and Chorizo Pie 13
Daly Dog, The 111
Cinema-style Nachos 95
Cinnamon Swirl Pancakes 194
Classic Double Cheeseburger 150
coleslaw, Traditional Coleslaw 143
Cottage Pie 33
cream/sour cream
Beef Burrito 30
Chicken Alfredo 170
Faddyjattys 34
That Pasta 178
crisps, Cheese and Onion Crisps 114
Crispy Chicken Fillet Roll 98
Crispy Shredded Mushrooms 110
Crispy Tikka Chicken Kebabs 90
Crispy Waffles 199

D
Daly Dog, The 111
Deadly Doughnuts 201
Dishy Hash Browns 102
Doner Kebab 83
doughnuts, Deadly Doughnuts 201
Durty Fries 149

E
eggs
Airfryer Omelette 58

Best Southern Fried Chicken, The 48
Breakfast Biscuits 204
Brownies 206
Cake in a Cup 205
Carbonara 182
Chicken Kiev 36
Chickpea Waffles 120
Cinnamon Swirl Pancakes 194
Crispy Chicken Fillet Roll 98
Crispy Waffles 199
Deadly Doughnuts 201
Epic Scramble 166
Fish and Chips 154
Fish Burger 156
Fruity and Fab French Toast 162
Perfect Poached Eggs 103
Po'boy 108
Red Velvet Breakfast Pancakes 196
Sausage and Egg Muffin From Scratch 101
Spice Bag Burger 70-2
Suppli 190
Swiss Roll Pancake 200
Epic Scramble 166

F
Faddyjattys 34
Fish and Chips 154
Fish Burger 156
Fruity and Fab French Toast 162

G
Garlic and Cheese Fries 65
garlic butter 36
Guacaholymoley 137

H
ham
Airfryer Omelette 58
On-the-pan Cheese Toastie 106

Prosciutto and Mozzarella
Pizza Wrap 186
Prosciutto-wrapped
Asparagus 172
see also bacon; pork
hazelnuts
Masso Mushrooms 165
Nuteile 208
herbs and spices 7
Homemade Biscoff Spread 209
Honey and Sriracha-glazed
Airfryer Brussels Sprouts 52

I

instant mash
Best Southern Fried
Chicken, The 48
Black Bean Crispy Chicken
73
Buffalo Fries 80
Chicken Kiev 36
Crispy Tikka Chicken
Kebabs 90
Po'boy 108
Sexy Spice Bag 63–4
Spice Bag Burger 70–2
Sweet and Sour Chicken 68
Veggie Fingers/Nuggets 53
Irish stout, Beef and Stout Stew
24

J

jalapeños
Chicken Enchiladas 14
Daly Dog, The 111
Durty Fries 149
Guacaholymoley 137
Mexican Chilli Bowl 25

kale, Krispy Kale 116
Katsu Curry 21
kiwis, Fruity and Fab French
Toast 162
Krispy Kale 116

L

leeks
Chicken and Leek Vol-au-
Vents 23
Chicken, Leek and Chorizo
Pie 13
Luscious Lasagne 176

M

Mac and Cheese 161
Masso Mushrooms 165
Melanzana alla Parmigiana 179
Mexican Chilli Bowl 25
mozzarella
Luscious Lasagne 176
Melanzana alla Parmigiana
179
Prosciutto and Mozzarella
Pizza Wrap 186
Prosciutto-wrapped
Asparagus 172
Suppli 190
muffins, Sausage and Egg
Muffin From Scratch 101
mushrooms
Airfryer Omelette 58
Chicken and Leek Vol-au-
Vents 23
Chicken Enchiladas 14
Chicken, Leek and Chorizo
Pie 13
Crispy Shredded
Mushrooms 110
Faddyjattys 34
Masso Mushrooms 165
Mushroom and Asparagus
Soup 124
Prosciutto and Mozzarella
Pizza Wrap 186
Spicy Cheesy Chicken
Calzones 184
Stroganoff Sauce 136
That Pasta 178
Veggie Pudding Stack 130

N

nachos, Cinema-style Nachos 95
New Yorker, The 107
Not Nuts Nuts 115
Not Szechuan Beef 84
Nuteile 208

O

omelette, Airfryer Omelette 58
On-the-pan Cheese Toastie 106

P

pancakes
Cinnamon Swirl Pancakes
194
Red Velvet Breakfast
Pancakes 196
Swiss Roll Pancake 200
panko breadcrumbs
Banging Blue Burger 146
Classic Double
Cheeseburger 150
Crispy Chicken Fillet Roll
98
Fish and Chips 154
Fish Burger 156
Katsu Curry 21
Suppli 190
Parmesan cheese
Aglio Olio Peperoncino 173
Carbonara 182
Cheesy Chickrizo Pasta 18
Chicken Alfredo 170
Chicken and Leek Vol-au-
Vents 23
Krispy Kale 116
Melanzana alla Parmigiana
179
Mushroom and Asparagus
Soup 124
Spag Bol 183
That Pasta 178
Tomato Bruschetta with
Balsamic Vinegar 187
passata
Chicken Enchiladas 14
Cottage Pie 33

Luscious Lasagne 176
Melanzana alla Parmigiana 179
Mexican Chilli Bowl 25
Not Szechuan Beef 84
Spag Bol 183
Suppli 190
pasta
    Aglio Olio Peperoncino 173
    Carbonara 182
    Cheesy Chickrizo Pasta 18
    Chicken Alfredo 170
    Luscious Lasagne 176
    Mac and Cheese 161
    Spag Bol 183
    That Pasta 178
pastrami
    New Yorker, The 107
    Rockin' Reuben Salad 119
peanut butter, Terrifically Tasty Beef Satay 10
peas
    Beef and Stout Stew 24
    Chicken Fried Rice 86
    Cottage Pie 33
    Me Ma's Chicken Curry 16
    Suppli 190
    Veggie Fingers/Nuggets 53
pepperoni, Airfryer Pizza Bagels 56
peppers
    Beef Burrito 30
    Black Bean Crispy Chicken 73
    Chicken Enchiladas 14
    Crispy Tikka Chicken Kebabs 90
    Faddyjattys 34
    Fish Burger 156
    Mexican Chilli Bowl 25
    Not Szechuan Beef 84
    Philly Cheese Steak 22
    Sexy Spice Bag 63–4
    Spice Bag Burger 70–2
    Super-speedy Spring Rolls 76–7
    Sweet and Sour Chicken 68

Perfect Chips 44
Perfect Poached Eggs 103
Philly Cheese Steak 22
pickles
    Airfryer Frickles 50
    New Yorker, The 107
    Rockin' Reuben Salad 119
    Sticky Chicken Burger 89
Po'boy 108
pork
    Sausage and Egg Muffin From Scratch 101
    see also bacon; ham
porridge oats
    Breakfast Biscuits 204
    Brownies 206
    Cake in a Cup 205
    Cinnamon Swirl Pancakes 194
    Crispy Waffles 199
    Deadly Doughnuts 201
    Nuteile 208
    Red Velvet Breakfast Pancakes 196
    Vegan Burgers 38
potatoes
    Beef and Stout Stew 24
    Bubble and Squeak 40
    Buffalo Fries 80
    Cheese and Onion Crisps 114
    Chicken, Leek and Chorizo Pie 13
    Cottage Pie 33
    Dishy Hash Browns 102
    Durty Fries 149
    Fish Burger 156
    Fish and Chips 154
    Garlic and Cheese Fries 65
    New Yorker, The 107
    Perfect Chips 44
    Sexy Spice Bag 63–4
    Spice Bag Burger 70–2
    Spicy Cheesy Chicken Calzones 184
    Veggie Fingers/Nuggets 53
    Veggie Pudding Stack 130
prawns, Po'boy 108

Prosciutto and Mozzarella Pizza Wrap 186
Prosciutto-wrapped Asparagus 172

R
Red Velvet Breakfast Pancakes 196
rice
    Beef Burrito 30
    Chicken Fried Rice 86
    Crispy Shredded Mushrooms 110
    Katsu Curry 21
    Me Ma's Chicken Curry 16
    Suppli 190
    Terrifically Tasty Beef Satay 10
rice noodles
    Curry Noodle Soup 122
    Super-speedy Spring Rolls 76–7
rice paper, Super-speedy Spring Rolls 76–7
Rockin' Reuben Salad 119

S
Sage and Onion Stuffing 41
sauces
    black bean sauce 73
    Burger Sauce 140
    Cheese Sauce 134
    enchilada sauce 14
    Guacaholymoley 137
    satay sauce 10
    sticky soy and ginger sauce 110
    Stroganoff Sauce 136
    sweet and sour sauce 68
    Tarty Sauce 141
sauerkraut, Rockin' Reuben Salad 119
Sausage and Egg Muffin From Scratch 101
Sexy Spice Bag 63–4
shopping list 6–7

soup
    Curry Noodle Soup 122
    Mushroom and Asparagus
        Soup 124
    Spicy Tomato Soup 127
Spag Bol 183
Spice Bag Burger 70–2
Spicy Cheesy Chicken Calzones
  184
Spicy Tomato Soup 127
spinach
    Cheesy Curry Beans on
        Toast 164
    Curry Noodle Soup 122
Sticky Chicken Burger 89
Stroganoff Sauce 136
stuffing, Sage and Onion
  Stuffing 41
Super-speedy Spring Rolls 76–7
Suppli 190
Sweet and Sour Chicken 68
sweetcorn
    Beef Burrito 30
    Buffalo Veggie Wrap 94
    Vegan Burgers 38
    Veggie Fingers/Nuggets 53
Swiss Roll Pancake 200

T

Tarty Sauce 141
Teriyaki Yuk Sung 74
That Pasta 178
tomatoes
    Airfryer Pizza Bagels 56
    Banging Blue Burger 146
    Crispy Chicken Fillet Roll
        98
    Guacaholymoley 137
    Luscious Lasagne 176
    Melanzana alla Parmigiana
        179
    On-the-pan Cheese Toastie
        106
    Po'boy 108
    Prosciutto and Mozzarella
        Pizza Wrap 186
    Spag Bol 183

Spicy Tomato Soup 127
    Tomato Bruschetta with
        Balsamic Vinegar 187
    see also passata
Traditional Coleslaw 143

V

Vegan Burgers 38
vegetables (mixed)
    Curry Noodle Soup 122
    Terrifically Testy Beef Satay
        10
Veggie Fingers/Nuggets 53
Veggie Pudding Stack 130

W

waffles, Crispy Waffles 199
wraps
    Beef Burrito 30
    Buffalo Veggie Wrap 94
    Chicken and Leek Vol-au-
        Vents 23
    Chicken Enchiladas 14
    Cinema-style Nachos 95
    Crispy Tikka Chicken
        Kebabs 90
    Faddyjattys 34
    Prosciutto and Mozzarella
        Pizza Wrap 186
    Spicy Cheesy Chicken
        Calzones 184

Y

yoghurt
    Brownies 206
    Crispy Tikka Chicken
        Kebabs 90
    Red Velvet Breakfast
        Pancakes 196
    Swiss Roll Pancake 200

Z

zero-sugar sodas
    Not Szechuan Beef 84
    Sweet and Sour Chicken 68
    Teriyaki Yuk Sung 74
    Terrifically Tasty Beef Satay
        10

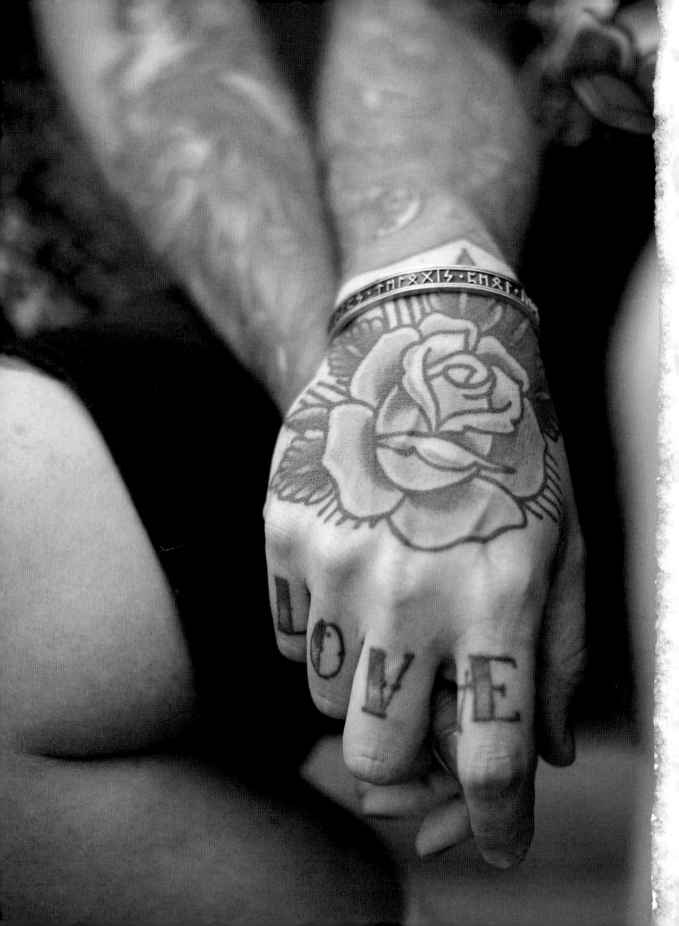